EARTH MEDICINE-
EARTH FOOD

EARTH MEDICINE–
EARTH FOOD

Plant Remedies, Drugs, and Natural Foods of the North American Indians

Revised and Expanded

MICHAEL A. WEINER

FAWCETT COLUMBINE · NEW YORK

EARTH MEDICINE, EARTH FOOD is an histori-
cal/anthropological guide to wild foods and herbal
remedies traditionally used by North American Indians. It is not intended to treat, diagnose or prescribe.
If you know or suspect you have a serious health problem, we suggest you consult a professional health
worker.

A Fawcett Columbine Book
Published by Ballantine Books

Copyright © 1972, 1980 by Michael A. Weiner

All rights reserved under International and Pan-American
Copyright Conventions. Published in the United States
by Ballantine Books, a division of Random House, Inc.,
New York, and simultaneously in Canada by Ramdom House of
Canada Limited, Toronto. Originally published in somewhat
different form by Macmillan Publishing Company in 1972. First
revised and expanded edition published in 1980.

Library of Congress Catalog Card Number: 90-82344

ISBN: 0-449-90589-6

Cover design by William G. Geller

Manufactured in the United States of America

First Ballantine Books Edition: January 1991

10 9 8 7 6 5 4 3 2 1

In memory of Ben Weiner
who first led me
to the woods.

To Rachel Weiner
who kept me
dry.

LIST OF ILLUSTRATIONS

CONTENTS

1. Earth Medicine

2. Earth Food

Part I

EARTH MEDICINE

INTRODUCTION TO THE REVISED AND EXPANDED EDITION

The Cherokee still preserve the custom of consecrating a family of their tribe to the priesthood, as the family of Levi was consecrated among the Jews.

John G. Bourke,
Medicine Men of the Apache (1891)

Spiritual Hedonism and the Search for Healing Plants

By drinking from too many wells, each of good water, we may confuse our bodies and wind up in worse shape than when we began. To arrive at the well of herbs and take them on a casual basis is inappropriate, both medically and spiritually. We may wish to open up our inner channels through acupuncture, massage, movement, and through the proper use of diet, including herbs. But approaching our spiritual source, the well of all cures, through our physical senses must be fulfilled by a spiritual offering, not merely the experience of a fleeting pleasure.

The Indian peoples who preceded us on this land were aware of this need to pay the "great creator" and they utilized herbs as one part of a greater healing totality. To strip herbs from their origins without appreciating the greater context from which they derive may effect temporary adjustments in our health without yielding the more lasting "cure."

Now it is true that d-tubocurarine, derived from the curare plant, will drastically relax your muscles whether you be a Brazilian Indian, an Alaskan Eskimo, or a concrete dweller, without any rituals whatever. So why bother studying various cultural beliefs surrounding herbal medicine when we can simply use those plants with known, established therapeutic actions? Simply because we, as spiritual physiological beings, benefit from learning

about healing rituals. By delving into the cultural beliefs of other peoples, we become more curious about our own. And by investigating our own ancestral health-codes, we may come to see the interconnections between all peoples, a worthy, unifying goal.

Just taking herbs whenever we feel like doing so while also dropping some vitamins, getting massaged, and so on, is a form of *spiritual hedonism* or *medical consumerism* disguised in the frock of seeking the gentler path.

We in the Western "alternative health" world seem to be sampling from *all* healing modes at once. Eclectic medicine would be appropriate if we limited ourselves to curing our ills. But so many of us seem to be wanting just *more* health or *better* health, an almost greedy desire to get the most for ourselves. While the native Americans also sought their health, we have no record of their having an obsession with healing.

In reading through the remedies that follow, be aware of the seriousness of the overall healing ceremonies that accompanied these cures. While the author has separated the herbal remedies from the cultures that gave them birth, a guide to more complete descriptions of the healing ceremonies and the healers themselves can be found in the bibliography. One manuscript in particular is representative of this aspect of Amerindian healing. This is the revised edition of James Mooney's 1891 work, entitled *The Swimmer Manuscript: Cherokee Sacred Formulas & Medicinal Prescriptions* (1929).

Cherokee Sacred Formulas and the Search for Disease Causation

While Cherokee beliefs regarding disease causation do not necessarily help us to heal our-

3

selves, they may not be any more "irrational" than many biochemical theories offered to us by the groping Western medical technicians.

If even in cases where the natural course and cause of events seems evident and obvious, a mythologic explanation may be advanced, what are we to expect when it becomes necessary to account for such mysterious, unexplainable, insidious changes of condition as those to which disease subjects our body and mind?

The man who but two or three days ago was a living image of both Hercules and Adonis, and who came home from the mountain carrying on his shoulder a tree trunk of formidable weight and dimension as lightly as if it were but a bark canoe, today lies prostrate, pain- and terror-stricken, with haggard looks and sallow complexion, suffering, panting, and grasping. . . .

The buxom woman, from whom last week a chubby, healthy baby boy "jumped down," as the Cherokee express it, is now suffering more than ever she did, and feels herself as being burned by a scorching internal fire. . . .

The sprightly baby, which ever since it moved was as alert and bustling as a young chipmunk or scampering squirrel, suddenly lapses into spasmodic convulsions, or lies motionless with haggard eyes as wide open as those of a terror-stricken rabbit. . . .

Why? For what reason?

When we think of how, in a civilized community, as soon as anything uncanny happens, as soon as the Awful Incomprehensible makes its presence felt, even the sophisticated lose their reasoning faculties and grasp at ridiculous explana-

tions and at impossible hopes, how can we scoff at the conclusions these poor people reach?

Cherokee "Reasons" for These Ills

The man who became ill so suddenly had had a quarrel a week or so ago with an ill-reputed medicine man, who told him, as they separated, that he would hear about him again. The wizard has shot an invisible flint arrowhead into his bowels.

The woman who had known the joys of such a happy delivery had not heeded the subsequent taboo prohibiting all warm food to anyone in her condition. That is why she is now being consumed by an internal fire.

The baby is now paying the penalty of his mother having partaken of rabbit meat during her pregnancy, six months or so ago. And that is why it is now assuming the cramped position, so reminiscent of the hunchback position of a squatting rabbit, or why its eyeballs are so dilated.

The Amerindians, often at war with one another, nevertheless shared many herbal remedies, if not beliefs. Where common tribal usages of herbs display a pattern, being recorded as employed by tribes in varying geographies, they have been selected for this compendium. Most plants have also appeared in later editions of the *U.S. Dispensatory* or the *National Formulary*, attesting to their efficacy. So, of the many hundreds of plants known to the American Indian healers, here you will find the safest, surest bets.

INTRODUCTION

Medical treatment is older than intelligence in man. The dog hunts the fields for his special grass medicine; the bear dresses the wound of her cub or fellow-bear with perhaps as much intelligence as primitive man observes in his empirical practice. Primitive man does not know why his medicine cures; he simply knows that it does cure.

Matilda Coxe Stevenson
"Ethnobotany of the Zuñi Indians"

Whereas modern man relies upon the drugstore, the early Indians who preceded us on this continent utilized the healing plants of the forests, deserts, and seashores. Although our prescription drugs are available in handy, colorful, even tasty, forms and all appear to be "factory made" or of synthetic chemical origin, over 25 percent of all prescriptions contain a drug from natural plant sources. The average physician in the United States still writes at least eight prescriptions daily for drugs of plant origin. In 1967, plant drugs accounted for more than 300 million dollars' worth of all pharmaceuticals used in the United States.

In an age of synthetics, nature still provides us with products that are widely used, simply because the complexity of the compounds in these plants would make the cost of laboratory synthesis too expensive.

When the early settlers first arrived in North America, many carried with them herbal remedies which were then commonly employed in Europe. They soon realized the problems involved in trying to keep fresh the dried plants arriving from across the Atlantic Ocean. Some then brought in seeds from Europe and planted their own herbal gardens. Others drank in the then limitless mystery and beauty of America and realized that the forests of the New World must hold many cures for their ills. But how were they going to learn which plant was useful for their specific problem? Many Europeans undoubtedly saw similarities between the useful plants of the Old World and those of America. These early observations probably led many desperately sick people to try the new plants in attempts to cure themselves. No doubt many died as a result of biting into a poisonous species.

The spirit that led the early settlers to try strange plants is to be admired. For, like some pharmaceutical laboratories of today, these early herbalists would experiment with almost every root they stumbled upon, hoping to find a cure for a severe illness. Some of their patients lived and were cured, others no doubt were not cured, and some died. If more patients were cured than not, the plant in question became a popular remedy. This method of trial and error, however, was too risky for some. More cautious settlers began to ask the native inhabitants of America—the Indians—to show them which plants were useful for curing sickness. Since the Indians were at first friendly to the newcomers, they showed them some of their healing plants. Soon many Indian medicine men were treating both whites and natives. One plant, the joe-pye weed, received its popular name from an Indian herbalist from New England who reportedly cured typhus with it by inducing profuse sweating. This plant was eventually admitted to the *United States Pharmacopoeia*, but for different medical purposes.

The remedies described in this book came to us through books and letters written *after* Europeans arrived in North America. We cannot safely say that all these plant remedies were derived solely from native Americans; many are probably derived from those settlers who were quick in adapting to their new environment. Indians sometimes borrowed remedies from the settlers and passed them along, so that eventually they became known as Indian remedies.

This book is essentially a translation of records of the Indians' plant medicine; it also includes the medicine of our grandfathers' physicians. These physicians learned about the medicinal uses of many plants from the Indians—but did they know which plants were of true medicinal value? This can be answered only by looking to the *U.S. Pharmacopoeia*, the *National Formulary*, and the

Dispensatory of the United States to see which of these early remedies became official drugs. If we recognize these reference works as the standard for all drugs used in American medical practice, then it becomes an easy task to evaluate the relative values of the plant medicines used by our grandfathers. If they were admitted to the *Pharmacopoeia* then, we might say, they are obviously valuable; but the evaluation is not this simple. What do we conclude about those plants which were admitted to these reference works but later withdrawn? Were they deleted because further experimentation proved they were dangerous or worthless? Or, were these once-popular remedies dropped because a synthetic drug replaced them, regardless of their usefulness? In this light it becomes extremely difficult to make a decision about the value of the plants described in the following pages. For this reason, I have decided to follow the presentation of the *Dispensatory of the United States*, which cites the uses to which drugs have been put without recommending them. In adopting this format, all usage is presented in the past tense. The information is presented without advocacy.

Indian remedies came to us from the writings of travelers, missionaries, soldiers, anthropologists, and botanists. The main source of information about plants used in American medical practice during the last century is Dr. C. F. Millspaugh, the botanist–physician who wrote the classic work *American Medicinal Plants* in 1887. In addition to discussing the most important medicinal plants of his time, he painted 180 original plates from living plants. Many of his fine illustrations are reproduced here. In addition, illustrations were also drawn from two nineteenth-century English editions on this subject; from Woodville's *Medical Botany* (1832) and from Bentley's *Medicinal Plants* (1880). That so many native American plants appear in these English works indicates how rapidly some Indian remedies were accepted.

Does the fact that our early physicians borrowed many remedies from Indian practitioners mean that the Indian was always correct in his choices? We cannot answer this question directly; we may only assume that the Indian was able to cure himself of many complaints and to alleviate the suffering of others. We must remember that the life expectancy of the early American Indian, as evaluated from bones that remain, was about thirty-seven years. Therefore, many illnesses common to older people were unknown or uncommon until the European came to this continent. Then, by virtue of contagion, and later by an "improved" standard of living, the Indian inherited many "new" illnesses with his increased life span. Some remedies described in this book, for example, the use of devil's club to cure diabetes, originated with the Indians of this century. Confronted with new medical problems, the Indian looked to the plants of his environment for cures right up to this century. But how did he learn which plants were valuable? How did the American Indian decipher the secrets of his plant environment?

The medicinal plant lore of most primitive peoples is founded on a local "doctrine of signatures." According to this theory, many medicinal plants exhibit clearly visible signs which indicate their uses. "Like cures like," and for every illness there exists a cure, goes the doctrine. Persons who ascribed to this idea held that the shape or color of particular plants pointed the way to cures. In most cases the American Indian interpreted this idea to mean that to eliminate worms they needed a plant that resembled a worm; for treating inflamed eyes they selected a flower that resembled the eye of a deer. The Hopi used plants which exude a milky juice to promote the secretion of milk in nursing women. Members of this tribe held that a gnarled piece of wood was important in the treatment of convulsions.

The "doctrine of signatures" was not limited to plants. The Hopi named a plant weasel medicine because it resembled that animal. They reasoned that since the weasel is able to dig through the ground very quickly, the plant named for him would speed childbirth, and they used this plant for that purpose.

The Indians were not the only ones to practice according to this doctrine. Both the early settlers, who were Europeans, and ancient practitioners of the Old World ascribed to the same idea. Thus, liverleaf was once popularly used to cure chronic hepatitis in Europe. To understand how some early herbalists decided to use this plant as a cure for liver disorders, you need only study the shape of the leaves (FIG. 1). Other examples of this doctrine are found throughout "Earth Medicine" and the clearest case is that of the herb St.-John's-wort, which is discussed under "Respiratory Problems."

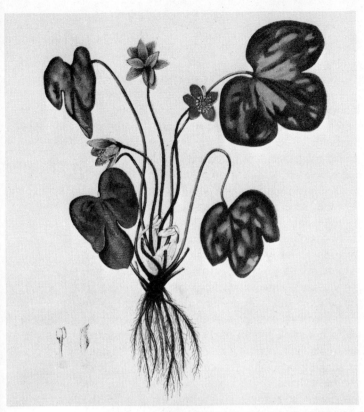

(FIG. 1) *LIVERLEAF: Some tribes practiced medicine according to the ancient "doctrine of signatures." The leaves of this plant, which look like the human liver, were used by early Europeans to treat liver disorders.*

Of course, not all tribes sought their cures through a doctrine of "like cures like." Some relied upon the supernatural, while others probably experimented with plants and learned by trial and error. After a good sniff and a little nibble, the Indian herbalist either accepted or rejected the plant in question. If he tried a poisonous variety and died, his fellow tribesmen never heard from him again. If a trial root, bark, or leaf cured an early practitioner, he either kept it to himself and became a renowned village "healer" or he passed his new knowledge on to the next unfortunate who showed outward signs of needing that particular plant remedy.

Not all questions concerning the value of some American Indian plant medicines remain unanswered. An early visitor to this continent reported that the Canadian Indian cured himself of smallpox by using a tea of the leaves of a little-known species, the bog-dwelling pitcher plant. Likewise, Cartier's men were cured of scurvy by drinking a tea of the bright green needles of vitamin-C-rich black spruce as given to them by a tribe of In-

dians. Also, long before a large American drug company marketed a laxative from the leaves of cascara sagrada, the Indians of northern California had been using it for the same effect. And, if we consider narcotics to be valuable drugs, it becomes remarkable that *Datura meteloides* was used in America for centuries before it was introduced for the same purpose in Europe. These examples and many others described in "Earth Medicine" will show that without the hardware common to our monolithlike laboratories the American Indian discovered and used many beneficial plant drugs. It is a fact that approximately one hundred and seventy drugs which are now, or were once, official in the *U.S. Pharmacopoeia* or the *National Formulary* were utilized by the Indians of North America. Further, hundreds of other plant medicines which have not become accepted in our official books on plant medicines were also used by the American Indian.

Not only was the American Indian adept at healing certain ailments with plants, but he was also ahead of his time in certain other areas of treatment. Most tribes practiced Crede's method of eliminating the afterbirth at least one hundred years before this procedure was published in a European medical journal. The Indians' ability to heal serious wounds was marveled at by even the most ardent Indian haters among the U.S. Cavalry; some of their methods are described under "Wounds."

The usual means of preparing various plants for internal use was in the form of a decoction. Plant parts were gathered in advance and dried before being boiled in water to make the medicinal teas. (The word *tea* is employed freely throughout this book and is meant to describe a boiled or steeped liquid preparation of various plant parts. It is not used to describe common tea, as we know it.) Generally, Indian herbal remedies were composed of one plant—sometimes two or three. Rarely do we find a record which indicates that many plants were combined to make a single medicine. An exception is found in a Mohegan recipe for a spring tonic. Twelve plants were steeped, and the resulting tea taken to awaken the spirit at the onset of spring.

These decoctions were often taken only once throughout the course of an illness and not repeated. Dosage usually consisted of about one pint of the medicinal tea. It is interesting to note that small amounts of a particular medicine were sometimes used for certain diseases, while large amounts of the same preparation were given for other troubles. For example, the Thompson Indians of British Columbia used a weak decoction of the wood of snowberry for washing babies, while a stronger decoction of the wood was used for treating sores.

All tribes certainly recognized that certain medicines might cure an ailment but harm the patient in other ways. These "side effects" were avoided by taking special precautions, such as abstaining from certain foods or liquids for several days following treatment.

In some cases plants that were safe to use in one state were deadly in others. This was the case with angelica (FIG. 2). The roots of this species were smoked with tobacco and even eaten as an emergency food after they had been dried but were poisonous when freshly dug. Certain Canadian tribes ate the fresh roots of this plant for suicidal purposes. Similarly, the Thompson Indians employed a decoction of the roots of baneberry as a cure for syphilis and rheumatism, but they were very cautious with the dosage because

(FIG. 2) ANGELICA: *The roots of this plant are poisonous when fresh and were used for suicidal purposes by certain Canadian tribes. In the dry state they lose this dangerous property. Arkansas Indians smoked the leaves with tobacco and even ate them when necessary.*

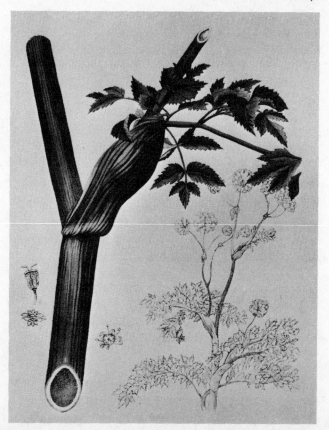

too strong a decoction sometimes resulted in death.

The American Indian was expert at gathering and utilizing the plants of his environment; he knew when plants were most potent and best suited for collection prior to being made into medicine. Alice Henkel, an American expert on medicinal plants, compiled extensive data on the collection and preservation of many species. Much of her information, no doubt, was gathered through several generations and originated to some extent with the native American. Generally, the roots of annual plants were dug before flowering, in the early spring, while those of biennial or perennial herbs were gathered in late fall when growth had ceased and the plant was storing its nutrients before winter. The object of gathering during certain seasons was to take the plant part when it was richest in medicinal properties. After the roots had been collected, they were cleaned by shaking or washing, then either dried for later use or utilized in the fresh state. If dried, the roots were sometimes sliced and exposed to the air on racks, but they were never placed in direct sunlight. Miss Henkel states that it generally takes from three to six weeks for roots to dry, depending on the weather and the nature of the plant.

If the bark was the part desired, it was gathered when it was most easily slipped from the trunk and branches, during the winter or early spring. The outer layer was generally removed first and the inner layer then collected for use. In some cases the inner layer, between the inner bark and the wood, known as the cambium layer, was utilized for medicine and also for food because it was often very rich in useful material.

Leaves were gathered before the time of blooming and were dried in the shade away from dampness. Some remedies specifically called for young leaves, while others referred to the use of mature leaves.

Flowers, which were not frequently employed in Indian medicine except for ceremonial concoctions, were gathered when they first opened and carefully prevented from withering by eliminating moisture. Fruits, such as berries, were gathered at maturity and, again, either utilized in the fresh state or preserved for later use. Seeds were generally collected before the seed pods opened.

Although the Indian did possess great knowledge about the edible and healing plants of his environment, it must be remembered that he did not possess a universal knowledge. This book was written because there is yet much to be relearned from the medicine of the American Indian. Yet, it must be remembered that the author does not ascribe to the concept of the "noble savage." True, the Indian did live in great harmony with his natural surroundings; but it is certainly not true that the Indian was a peaceful man who merely communed with nature and enjoyed living with his fellow Indians. Many cases of savagery among the Indians themselves are documented. The enclosed illustration of a necklace of human fingers (FIG.3) was found by John G. Bourke, a captain in the U.S. Third Cavalry. This relic belonged to a Cheyenne medicine man and consisted of the fingers of Indians of hostile tribes. They had been carefully dissected and preserved in the form shown and were worn as a show of prowess. This is not the only record of intertribal hostility. Shoshoni scouts who accompanied U.S. troops on their terribly destructive raid of the Cheyenne at Powder River in Wyoming in 1876 discovered a buckskin bag which contained the hands of many of their own papooses and, in Bourke's words, they "danced and wailed all night, and then burned the tearful evidence of the loss sustained by their people."

These few examples of savagery are certainly not worse than the countless atrocities committed by other peoples of the world. I merely introduce them as evidence so that we may avoid the school

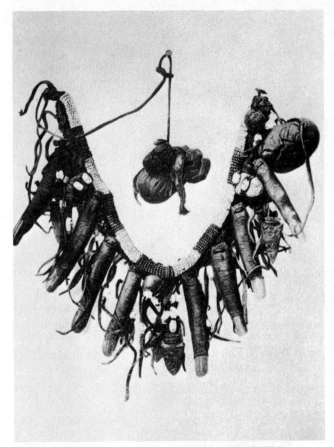

(FIG. 3) *NECKLACE OF HUMAN FINGERS: This trophy, which belonged to a Cheyenne, consisted of the fingers of Indians belonging to hostile tribes.*

of thought which holds that all American Indians had divine knowledge and therefore possessed a perfect understanding of the plants of their environment. We must read their remedies and remember that while some were no doubt useful, others were derived by fancy.

ABORTION

✌ ABORTIFACIENTS

Abortion was practiced only by tribes who were in contact with the whites. This was the case because half-breed babies were usually much larger than pure Indian babies, which created great difficulties in delivery, often endangering the mother's life. Abortion agents were not limited to plants. In some tribes the woman's abdomen was delivered a powerful blow, and in others slippery elm sticks were inserted into the cervix. Some plants which were used to induce abortion (termed abortifacients) follow.

✌ COTTON (FIG.4)

Among the Alabama and Koasati tribes a tea made of cotton roots boiled in water was taken to ease labor. It was thought that this decoction aided contractions in childbirth and that in high dosages it would induce abortion.

In 1840, a French writer, Bouchelle, reported that the root bark was widely used by Negro slaves in America to induce abortions. The root bark of this plant was officially recognized in the *U.S. Pharmacopoeia* for its effects on the uterine organs; for this reason it is possible that the abortifacient properties ascribed to cotton root bark by the Indian tribes listed above may be actual rather than imagined.

Laboratory studies of lower animals indicate that the root acts in a manner similar to that of ergot, though it is much less potent, and that it stimulates the uterus and causes contractions. Interestingly, the root bark is very rich in vitamin E.

The bark of cotton root, when collected for medicinal purposes, was gathered before frost set in, sometimes as late as December. The roots were washed in water, and the bark was removed and dried.

The cotton plant belongs to the mallow family and ranges between one and four feet in height.

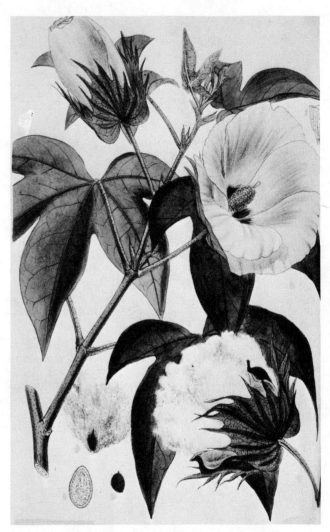

(FIG. 4) COTTON: *A tea made of the root bark was used by several tribes to ease labor in childbirth and to induce abortion.*

The leaves are composed of three to five sharply pointed lobes. The flowers are white when they first open but become purple on the second day. The oval cotton bolls are green at first but turn brown as they mature, eventually bursting open and exposing the fiber within—the cotton of commerce.

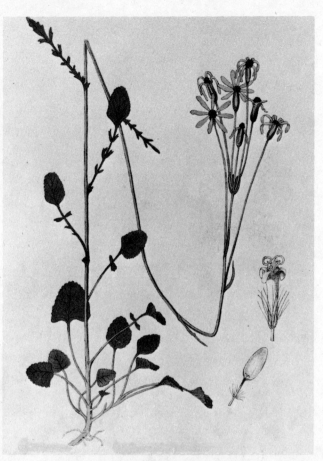

(FIG. 5) GOLDEN RAGWORT: *Several tribes referred to this herb as squawweed and used it extensively in treating problems associated with the female reproductive organs.*

～§ AMERICAN MISTLETOE

A tea was made from the leaves of the American mistletoe plant—which is parasitic on oaks and other trees of northern California—by various Indian tribes of Mendocino County. Taken in large quantities, it was said to cause abortion. Dr. W. H. Long, who may have first learned of the plant's use from the Indians, recommended it for use in domestic medicine because of its action on the uterus and for its ability to stop bleeding following parturition. Clinically, it has been shown that an extract of mistletoe causes an increase in uterine contractions and an increase in blood pressure when injected into the blood stream. A case of poisoning from eating the berries of this plant was recorded in Tennessee at the turn of the century.

～§ FLATSPINE RAGWEED

The Zuñi Indians of western New Mexico boiled the whole flatspine ragweed plant in water and drank the resulting tea to promote menstruation. They believed that if taken in large doses, this infusion could produce abortion. This weedy plant is found in moist soil from Saskatchewan to British Columbia and south to Texas. It looks similar to the great ragweed but has long, flat, straight spines on burrlike cones beneath the flower stalks.

～§ GOLDEN RAGWORT (FIG.5)

Golden ragwort was named squawweed by several tribes who utilized it extensively in problems associated with the female reproductive organs and to speed childbirth. The Catawba Indians, native to the region now defined as North Carolina, drank a tea prepared from the entire plant steeped in water. The ragwort has been used as a substitute for ergot and even as an antidote to poison-tipped arrows. Although pharmacologists have not reported any uterine effects, the plant does contain an essential oil, inuline, and the alkaloids senecine and senecionine, which are poisonous to livestock.

✑ TANSY (FIG.6)

Tansy was utilized medicinally by the Indians after being introduced to North America from Europe. In England, tansy was officially used to induce menstruation, while in America the Catawbas utilized a tea made from the entire plant for the same purpose and to induce abortion. Obviously, this tribe borrowed the application of tansy from the early white settlers.

As with most drugs, individual sensitivities may vary, and several fatal cases of poisoning from tansy tea have been recorded in the medical literature.

Other plants which were employed for their abortifacient properties and which will be treated in greater detail later on include sweet flag and Seneca snakeroot. The root of sweet flag was boiled in water and drunk by Indians in Montana to bring about abortion, while the bark of Seneca snakeroot was boiled and the resulting tea drunk for the same purpose by members of the Ottawa and Chippewa tribes. In domestic American practice, some women took pennyroyal leaf tea with brewer's yeast to induce abortion.

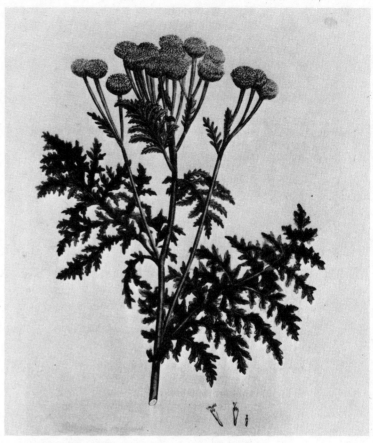

(FIG. 6) TANSY: *Soon after its introduction to America from Europe, the Catawbas utilized a tea prepared from this herb to induce abortion.*

ANTISEPTICS

AMERICAN MOUNTAIN ASH (FIG.7)

A small, smooth tree, the American mountain ash was formerly utilized in American medicine for the astringent, antiseptic properties of the inner bark. The bark of a European relative was used for fevers, and it is surprising that there is no record of Indian usage for this indigenous species. It is included here because it was employed in domestic medicine, which sometimes drew heavily on American Indian remedies. The brilliant red berries contain ascorbic acid and have been eaten to cure scurvy. As a tea, the berries yield an astringent liquid which was employed as a rectal wash for piles.

This smooth-barked tree occurs in swamps or moist grounds from Newfoundland south to North Carolina. It rarely exceeds thirty feet in height and has alternate leaves, each with eleven to seventeen lance-shaped, pointed leaflets.

The small white flowers appear in dense clusters about May or June and are followed in the fall by large, bright-red berries which are a favored food of many birds. Mountain ash also grows well on hilltops and rocky regions where fresh, cold spring water is absorbed by the roots. The sight of this tree, with its fernlike leaves and brilliant berries, is not easily forgotten.

BUTTERCUP (FIG.8)

All members of the genus *Ranunculus* are relatively poisonous and were generally applied externally. The Illinois Indians pulverized the root and, after soaking it in warm water, applied the wash to wounds and cuts. This genus was also

(FIG. 7) AMERICAN MOUNTAIN ASH: *The inner bark of this small tree was steeped in hot water and the resulting solution widely used as an antiseptic wash.*

(FIG. 8) BUTTERCUP: *The Illinois and other tribes pulverized the root, and after soaking it in warm water, applied the wash on wounds, cuts, etc.*

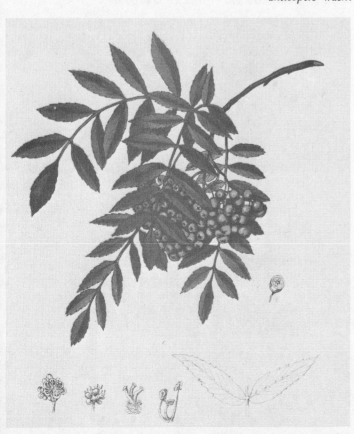

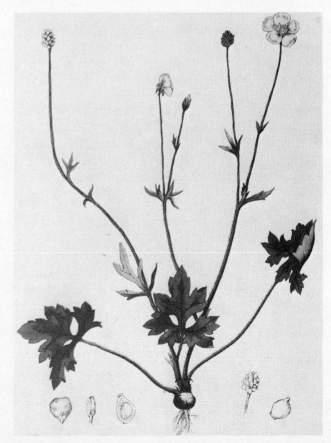

known to the ancient physicians; the blistering properties were described in Gerarde's *Herbal*: "Cunning beggars do use to stampe the leaves and lay it unto their legs and arms, which causeth such filthy ulcers as we daily see (among such wicked vagabondes), to moove the people the more to pittie."

A European variety of buttercup (*R. bulbosus*) was official in the *U.S. Pharmacopoeia* from 1820 to 1882 when it was used in American medicine as a counterirritant, to promote blistering of pimples, etc.

It was reported in 1887 that "violent attacks of epilepsy are recorded as having been induced by this plant, a sailor who inhaled the fumes of the burning plant was attacked with this disease for the first time in his life, it returned again in two weeks, passed into cachexia, nodous gout, headache, and terminated in death." This is interesting because it is reported that the Montagnais Indians of Newfoundland and Nova Scotia crushed and inhaled the vapor of a related species (*R. acris*) to cure headache.

ALPINE FIR

The gummy exudate which appears on the bark of the alpine fir was soaked in water until soft and then applied to wounds as an antiseptic by the Blackfoot Indians. The same tribe burned the needles for incense or prepared them as a tea for colds.

SWEET GUM (FIG. 9)

The balsam from sweet gum bark was first entered in the *U.S. Pharmacopoeia* in 1926 and is still officially recognized as being an antiseptic agent. This large tree has long been utilized in America for its healing properties. The Mississippi Choctaws applied hot water that had been boiled with the leaves of sweet gum directly on wounds, while the Choctaws of Bayou Lacomb combined the boiled roots with a decoction of pennywort roots and applied the wash to the injured area. The expert Virgil J. Vogel states in his book *American Indian Medicine* that an early visitor to America by the name of Bossu observed wild animals as they cured their wounds by rubbing against the fresh balsam of a sweet gum tree.

The tall forest dweller is one of the most beau-

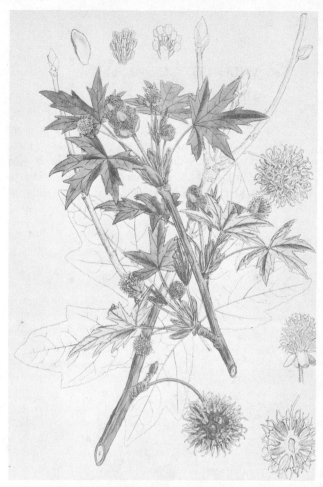

(FIG. 9) SWEET GUM: *The balsam from the bark of this tall forest dweller has long been used in America for its healing properties.*

tiful of native American trees. It sometimes attains a height of one hundred and fifty feet and is abundant in the low woods of the southeastern United States, occurring less frequently as far north as Connecticut. It grows straight and has very rough bark and short gray branches with corky ridges. The leaves are fragrant when bruised, occur alternately, and are star-shaped, with five lobes. The tree shows a hanging, thorny, ball-shaped fruit that contains many small seeds which are favored by birds. In the rain, the leaves look like glass stars with drops of silver falling from their points. The balsam occurs as a result of injury to the tree. To stimulate the tree to secrete this healing substance, the bark must be bruised or punctured by mechanical means.

The illustrated species, *Oriental Liquidambar*, is very similar to the American variety, differing only in the size of the fruit and the smoothness of the leaves.

WILD INDIGO (FIG.10)

The Mohegan tribe steeped the wild indigo root in water and applied the resulting liquid externally to wounds as an antiseptic wash. The Meskwakis utilized a variety of this plant (false indigo) for the same purpose. This herb was official in the *U.S. Pharmacopoeia* from 1831 to 1842 when it was used for its stimulant, astringent,

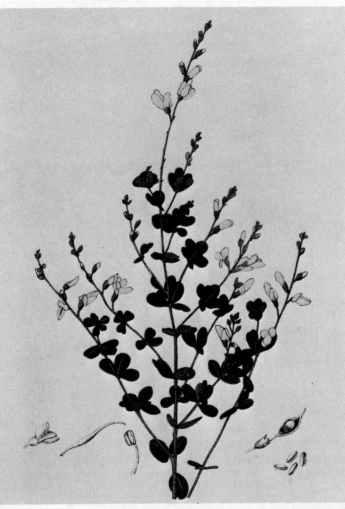

(FIG. 10) *WILD INDIGO: The Mohegans steeped the root in water and applied the resulting liquid externally to wounds as an antiseptic wash.*

and antiseptic properties. It was then applied to sores, skin ulcers, and eczema.

This slender, bushy branching herb grows two or three feet high and is found on dry land from Maine to Minnesota, south to Florida and Louisiana. From June to September it bears many canary yellow flowers about a half-inch long. Farmers once used this plant as a fly repellent for their horses by tying branches of it to the harness.

WHITE OAK

The majestic white oak tree was primarily utilized in Indian medicine to cure diarrhea and piles and is treated in more detail under these categories. The inner bark contains powerful antiseptic and astringent properties and was widely used for these purposes in American medicine. This bark layer, usually derived from trees between ten and twenty-five years old, is collected during the spring when it contains the greatest amount of tannic acid.

PIÑON

The piñon is one of the important edible plants of the Southwest. The nuts which appear inside the pine cones are collected in the late fall by the Navajos and other tribes. The Zuñi Indians prepared an antiseptic dusting power by drying and then pulverizing the resinous gum.

The piñon, which rarely exceeds fifty feet in height, grows on mesas in the Southwest. It is very abundant on the rim of the Grand Canyon and in the vicinity of Santa Fe, New Mexico. It shows short, brittle needles in clusters of two and three. The brittle wood has a smell of beeswax, is soft and light, and is sometimes used as fuel and for fence posts.

PLANTAIN (FIG.11)

The Indians named the common plantain white man's foot in reference to its trait of growing in the footsteps of the white man. That is, the plant was commonly introduced wherever a settlement was developed. It was used by the Shoshoni Indians, who heated the leaves and applied them in a wet dressing for wounds. The leaves were employed in early American medicine as an antidote to the effects of bites of venomous reptiles and insects, while the seeds were used as a worm remedy.

Boerhaave, an eighteenth-century European botanist, recommended plantain leaves bound to

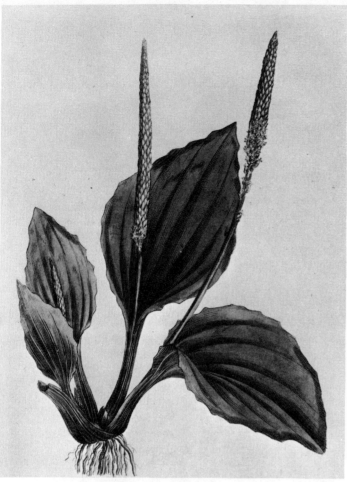

(FIG. 11) *PLANTAIN: The Shoshoni Indians heated the leaves and applied them in a wet dressing for wounds.*

aching feet to relieve the pain and fatigue of long hikes.

The Latin name, *plantago*, refers to the leaves which are shaped like the sole of a foot. This perennial herb is found in waste places throughout North America and is especially abundant in northern regions.

ᴇᵹ VALERIAN

The roots of the strong-smelling herb valerian were an essential drug in the medicine bags of the early Thompson Indian warriors who made sev-eral different preparations of it for wounds. Fresh roots were pulverized between stones and applied directly to the injured area, while the dried roots were employed as an antiseptic powder. The fresh leaves were sometimes chewed until they were moist and then applied to cuts and wounds.

The Thompson tribe of British Columbia probably discovered this species' value by trial and error long before the coming of the European. It is a well-known fact that some Indian groups had been using antiseptics before the time of Lister.

American valerian is native to southern Canada and ranges south to the Rocky Mountain region of New Mexico.

A related species of valerian (V. *officinalis*) was long used in European medicine where the plant was a native, and is even now cultivated in Holland, England, and Germany. It is employed as an antispasmodic and sedative in epilepsy and other nervous disorders. European valerian is very interestingly described in Woodville's *Medical Botany*, published at London in 1832:

> Its antispasmodic powers are very well established, and I trust to many of the reports that have been given of its efficacy; and if it has sometimes failed, I have just now accounted for it, adding only this, that it seems to me, in almost all cases, it should be given in larger doses than is commonly done. On this footing, I have frequently found it useful in epileptic, hysteric, and other spasmodic affections . . . the root, in substance, is most effectual, and is usually given in powder from a scruple to a dram: its unpleasant flavour may be concealed by a small addition of mace. A tincture of Valerian in proof spirit, and in volatile spirit, are ordered in the London Pharmacopoeia.

Even though the Thompson Indians employed the root of American valerian for antiseptic purposes, the European variety is considered to be an effective anticonvulsant. We see here an example of two cultures that were worlds apart that have discovered and utilized the plants of their environment.

APHRODISIACS

The excitement of one's sexual desire is a matter subject to one's whims and fortune. As with most subjective experiences the desire for sexual intercourse can be stimulated by most anything, depending on one's past experiences and the circumstance of the moment. The American Indian generally recognized the effects of sweet-scented flowers, charms, and rituals and employed them in the course of puberty rites, courtship, and marriage. A detailed account of several plants used in love potions comes to us from the lore of the Meskwakis as recorded by Huron H. Smith. This tribe lives in Wisconsin and is a division of the Fox clan. Their true Indian name is *Mĕshkwa Kihŭg*, which means "red earth people." This signifies the type of earth from which they believe they were created.

ᴥ JOE-PYE WEED

Although the joe-pye weed was named for an Indian doctor who reputedly cured typhus with it, the Meskwaki Indians considered it "a love medicine to be nibbled when speaking to women when they are in the wooing mood." Another name by which this plant is commonly referred to is purple boneset. This species, which belongs to the composite family, grows between three and ten feet high. It is composed of solid stems that are marked with purple at the point of leaf attachment. The leaves are usually in whorls of three to six and are coarsely serrated. When bruised, the plant emits a vanillalike odor. The flowers are elongated, white to pinkish or purple, and very numerous. The plant blooms between July and October and is found in moist soil from New Brunswick to Manitoba and south to Texas and South Carolina.

ᴥ RED AND BLUE LOBELIAS (FIG.12)

The Meskwakis also used the red and blue lobelias as love medicines. The roots of both were finely ground and secretly put into the food eaten

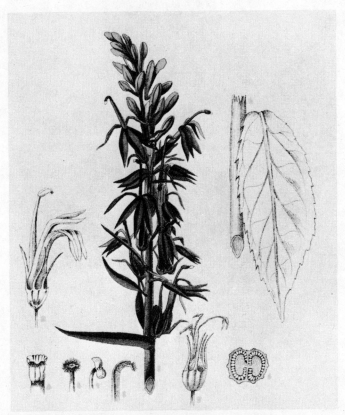

(FIG. 12) CARDINAL FLOWER: *The roots of this and of the blue lobelia were finely ground together and secretly put into the food eaten by an arguing couple to bring them together in love.*

by an arguing couple. This tribe believed that the use of this preparation "averts divorce and makes the pair love each other again."

ᴥ GINSENG (FIG.13)

The Meskwakis engaged in gathering ginseng as did many other tribes, who used it as a normal remedy, not ascribing it the magical powers believed inherent in the plant by the Chinese, French, and English. Trade was especially brisk in ginseng during the sixteenth century, and sometimes entire Indian villages engaged in digging out this root. In the 1790s the root was selling for as high as one dollar a pound, while more than one hundred years later it was bringing a commercial price of five dollars a pound. Some Chinese value the plant as a panacea (the shape of the root being most important to them). One small piece that looks like a man may bring a higher price than an entire bale. Before World War I, ginseng was one of the chief money-making crops in America, exports in 1906 amounting to 160,949 pounds which was then valued at $1,175,844.

This species, which is native to North America, was most frequently found growing in the moist soil of hardwood forests from Quebec to Ontario and south to the mountains of Georgia and Arkansas. Since it was overharvested, the plant is no longer easily found growing wild but is cultivated in artificial shade. Ginseng is an erect perennial herb which grows from eight to fifteen inches high and bears three leaves, each consisting of five thin, ovate leaflets which are pointed at the apex, the margins being toothed. During July and August, six to twenty greenish yellow flowers become apparent, which are soon followed by bright crimson berries.

The Meskwakis prepared a love potion consisting of ginseng root, mica, gelatin, and snake meat. It was used by their women to find a mate, and

(FIG. 13) GINSENG: *An ingredient in a Meskwaki love potion.*

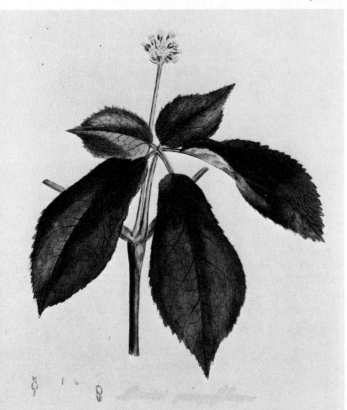

in the words of a Meskwaki, it is "a bagging agent women . . . use when they get a husband."

Among the Pawnee Indians ginseng was combined with three other plants (wild columbine, cardinal flower, and carrot-leaved parsley) to make a powerful love charm. As we learn from M. R. Gilmore, the anthropologist, when the suitor added hairs "obtained by stealth through the friendly offices of an amiably disposed third person from the head of the woman who was desired, she was unable to resist the attraction and soon yielded to the one who possessed the charm."

❧ DAYFLOWER

The use of love potions was not limited to the Meskwakis. The Navajos of the Southwest prepared an infusion of the dayflower which was drunk by aged men and women to increase their potency. As a testament to its usefulness, this tribe also gave the same preparation to their stud animals.

❧ LUPINE

The same tribe employed the lupine as a remedy for sterility and also believed that it favored the birth of female offspring if it was taken for several days preceding conception. As a sidenote, the word *lupinus* means "wolves" in Latin.

❧ WILD COLUMBINE

Omaha and Ponca men used the seeds of wild columbine as an aphrodisiac. Again, Gilmore wrote the story first:

For use as a love charm the pulverized seeds are rubbed in the palms, and the suitor contrives to shake hands with the desired one, whose fancy it is expected will thus be captivated. Omaha girls were somewhat in fear of the plant because of this supposed property and because, further, too strong a whiff of the odor was thought to cause nosebleed. On this account Omaha swains took delight in playfully frightening girls by suddenly thrusting some of the powder under their noses.

ASTHMA

SKUNK CABBAGE

The foul-smelling swamp dweller skunk cabbage was utilized by the Winnebago and Dakota tribes to stimulate the removal of phlegm in asthma. The rootstock was official in the *U.S. Pharmacopoeia* from 1820 to 1882 when it was employed in respiratory and nervous disorders and in rheumatism and dropsy.

MULLEIN (FIG.14)

The common pasture weed mullein was introduced from Europe where it had long been used as a medicinal plant. Evidently, the Indians learned from the early settlers that it was useful in treating respiratory problems because many

(FIG. 14) *MULLEIN: Several tribes smoked the leaves of this European pasture weed to relieve the symptoms of asthma.*

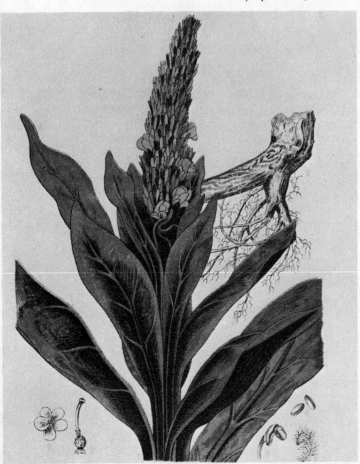

tribes reportedly employed the plant in a variety of treatments. The Menominees smoked the pulverized, dried root for respiratory complaints, while the Forest Potawatomis, the Mohegans, and the Penobscots smoked the dried leaves to relieve asthma. Since the American Indian did not often distinguish between the various respiratory ailments, such as bronchitis, asthma, and coughs, it is easy to comprehend how this velvety-textured weed came to be used for each of the above conditions. The literature on the Catawba Indians mentions another preparation, a sweetened syrup made from the boiled root, which they gave to their children for coughs.

Dr. Millspaugh noted that mullein was principally used around 1887 to relieve painful, phlegmy coughs. He also described a "cure" for hemorrhoids that consisted of a fatty oil which appeared after the bottled flowers were allowed to set in the sun.

By 1913, the plant had become extremely popular in America for treating coughs and inflamed conditions of the mucous membrane lining the throat. The corolla of the golden yellow flowers were gathered when they were fully opened and brought a wholesale price of seventy to eighty cents a pound. The blossoms are described as having the odor of honey and an equally sweet taste.

The erect stem of this weed rises to a maximum height of seven feet and has thick, rough velvety leaves arranged alternately until they reach the long, dense spike of yellow flowers. Mullein thrives in abandoned grass fields, and flowers from July to September.

INDIAN TOBACCO (FIG.15)

Indian tobacco was employed by several Indian tribes for various purposes, but it was not until the late eighteenth century that Indian tobacco first became a popular asthma remedy in American medicine. There appears to be some validity to this usage because the alkaloids present

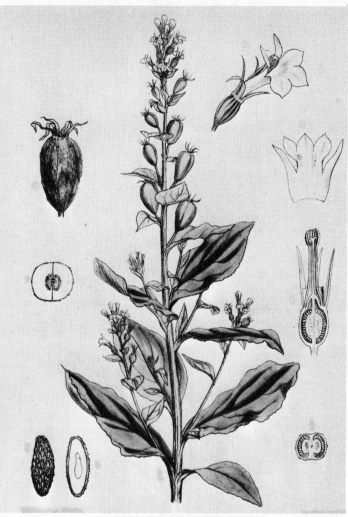

(FIG. 15) *INDIAN TOBACCO: Borrowed from the Indians, this plant became a popular asthma remedy in domestic American medicine. It is presently used in a number of antismoking preparations.*

in the leaves of this species have been utilized in medicines to stimulate the removal of phlegm from the respiratory tract. When chewed, the leaves induce headache, vomiting, and nausea. When too much of the plant has been ingested, coma and death have resulted. Like nicotine, the alkaloid lobeline first acts as a stimulant and then as a depressant to the autonomic nervous system. It also stimulates the vomiting center and in high dosage acts like curare, paralyzing muscular action. The *Dispensatory of the United States* says: "Its most important use in medicine is as a nauseating expectorant in bronchitis . . .

[and] large doses will sometimes cause complete cessation of the asthmatic paroxysms."

Indian tobacco is presently the subject of intensive research. The alkaloid lobeline, which it contains, is being used in a number of antismoking preparations, and scientists are attempting to cultivate the plant on a wide scale.

Indian tobacco is distinguished by its violet to whitish flowers which have oval bases that become swollen and hollow as the fruits develop. It is a branching annual herb from one to three feet in height and has numerous lance- or oval-shaped leaves from one to two and one-half inches long. The flowers appear in clusters at the branch tips between July and October. It is indigenous to the eastern and central United States and Canada.

JIMSON WEED

The extensive history and a catalog of Indian usage of the medicinally potent jimson weed is treated under "Narcotics and Mind-Altering Plants." At this point it may be interesting to note that in the early 1900s, the leaves of jimson weed were employed in the form of cigarettes and were smoked for asthma.

A word of caution for those who decide to experiment with the leaves without first calculating the hazards: DON'T! This member of the nightshade family contains atropine, which has caused poisoning and death in high dosage. Without belaboring the issue, I direct the interested reader to "Narcotics and Mind-Altering Plants" for the complete story of this deadly but intriguing plant.

Other plants which have been used with some reported success in asthma include evergreen sumac, the leaves of which were smoked; dragonroot, which was chewed; and the vine trumpet honeysuckle, which was dried and smoked.

Finally, it is worth listing yerba santa, which was smoked as a remedy for asthma and colds by the Indians of Mendocino County, California. (The medical and folk usage of this species is detailed under "Respiratory Problems" and is also briefly discussed under "Mouthwash.")

BACKACHE

ARNICA

The Catawba Indians utilized a tea of arnica roots for treating back pains. The dried flowerhead of European arnica has been in use in Europe since the sixteenth century largely as an application for bruises and sprains. The word *arnica* is thought to be derived from a Greek word for a sheep's skin. This reference to the softness of the leaves fails to suggest the bitter crystalline principle, arnicin, which is contained within and which exerts tonic, stimulant, and irritant effects.

The *Dispensatory of the United States* (22d ed.) states that this drug can be dangerous if taken internally and that it has caused severe and even fatal poisoning. The plant has been used in Europe for nervous disorders and appears to have been utilized in American domestic medicine primarily as a wash to treat sprains and bruises. European arnica has been official in the *U.S. Pharmacopoeia* from the early 1800s through 1960, again being used for sprains and bruises.

GENTIAN (FIG.16)

The Catawba Indians steeped the roots of American gentian in hot water and applied the resulting liquid on aching backs. European gentian, which is chemically similar, has long been used as a bitter digestive tonic. As illustrated, this European variety has yellow flowers, while the American variety shows blue flowers. Gentiana is named for Gentius, a King of Illyria who recognized the tonic properties of this plant. Gentian appears in the early Greek and Arabic herbals and was known to Pliny and Dioscorides. During the Middle Ages, it was also commonly employed as a medicine. The European species (*G. lutea*), which is illustrated, was official in the *U.S. Pharmacopoeia* from 1820 to 1955, when it was used as a gastric stimulant.

American gentian grows in the swampy area from Virginia to Florida. It has a simple, erect stem that grows between eight and ten inches

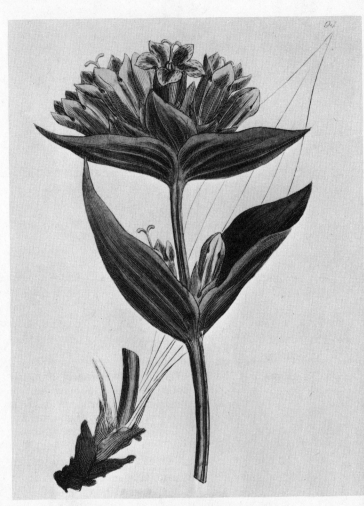

(FIG. 16) GENTIAN: *The Catawba Indians steeped the roots of American gentian in hot water and applied the resulting liquid on aching backs.*

high and bears opposite, ovate-lance–shaped leaves and pale blue flowers which appear from September to December.

HORSEMINT (FIG.17)

The Catawba tribe crushed and steeped fresh horsemint leaves in cold water and drank the infusion to allay the pain of backache. Other tribes employed horsemint for fever, inflammation, and chills. In American medicine of the nineteenth century, the oil derived from horsemint leaves was rubbed on the skin to promote sweating in typhus fever and rheumatism.

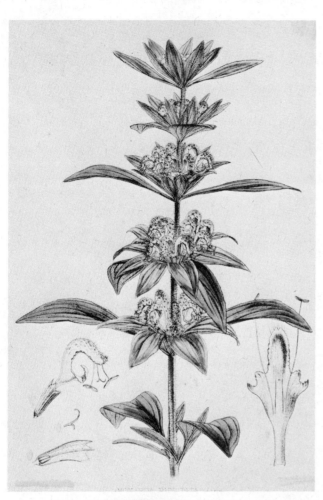

(FIG. 17) HORSEMINT: *The Catawbas crushed and steeped the fresh leaves in cold water and drank the infusion to allay the pain of backache.*

The leaves and flowering tops were official in the *U.S. Pharmacopoeia* from 1820 to 1882 and were used in rheumatism and as a digestive aid. Monarda oil and thymol are derived from the leaves. The latter derivative is an effective hookworm remedy, but must be ingested in such large doses that it is dangerous and frequently fatal.

ᴈᵹ SPIKENARD (FIG.18)

The aromatic herb spikenard was a popular remedy among several tribes of American Indians.

The Potawatomis prepared a poultice of the pulverized root for swellings and inflamed conditions, while the Shawnees applied spikenard for chest pains. The Ojibwa tribe combined the pounded roots with wild ginger and applied the mash as a wet dressing for broken bones. The Cherokees drank a tea of the roots for backache, and this remedy was soon adopted by the early settlers of the Great Smoky mountains.

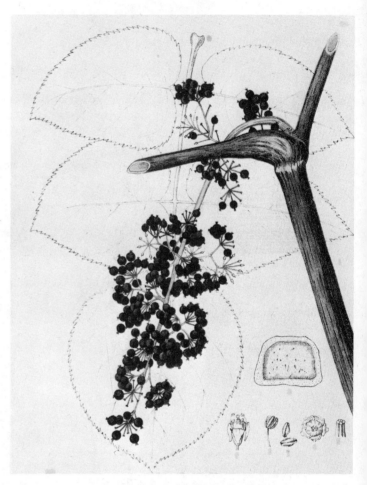

(FIG. 18) SPIKENARD: *The Cherokees drank a tea prepared from the roots for backache; this remedy was soon adopted by the early settlers of the Great Smoky Mountains.*

In the later part of the nineteenth century, the pulverized root was employed in domestic medicine for coughs, asthma, and rheumatism. Spikenard contains a saponin named aralin. The root was official in the *National Formulary* from 1916 to 1965 and was utilized in rheumatism and for skin problems.

This plant, which grows to a height of about six feet, exhibits several wide stems which bear large, alternate leaves. The small greenish flowers are borne on umbels and the small reddish purple fruits give the plant a striking appearance. Spikenard is indigenous to the eastern United States and Canada, west to Minnesota and Missouri. The roots and rhizomes are gathered in late summer and fall and cut lengthwise to facilitate drying.

BLISTERS

PIPSISSEWA (FIG.19)

The generic name of the pipsissewa, *Chimaphila*, was formed from two Greek words for "winter" and "friend." To draw out blisters, the Mohegans and the Penobscots, both tribes of the Northeast, steeped the plant in warm water and applied the liquid externally. The Thompson Indians of British Columbia pulverized the entire plant when fresh and applied the mass in a wet dressing to swellings of the lower legs and feet. Pipsissewa was used by other tribes as an internal medicine—to induce sweating, for rheumatism, for backache, etc.; however, the *Dispensatory of the United States* states that this plant has no medicinal properties.

(FIG. 19) PIPSISSEWA: *To draw blisters the Mohegans and the Penobscots steeped this small herb in warm water and applied the liquid externally.*

The plant was once a very popular home remedy among the early settlers of this country, especially the Pennsylvania Germans who used it as a tea to induce sweating. It was official in the *U.S. Pharmacopoeia* from 1820 through 1916 when it was employed for its astringent or tissue-drying properties.

This small member of the wintergreen family seldom exceeds one foot in height. Its shining, bright green leaves are broad at their tips and from one to two and one-half inches long. Pipsissewa thrives in dry woods and bears white or pinkish flowers in a small cluster at the end of a tall, erect stem.

SUNFLOWER (FIG.20)

The Ojibwa Indians crushed the root of the sunflower between stones and applied the mash in a wet dressing for drawing blisters.

(FIG. 20) SUNFLOWER: *The Ojibwa Indians crushed the root of this plant between stones and applied the mash in a wet dressing to draw blisters.*

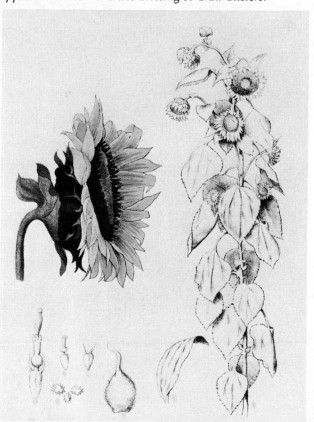

Although no other Indian medicinal uses for this species are recorded, a near relative, the common sunflower, is a widely used economic plant. Native to America, it is also grown for its sunflower oil in Russia, Bulgaria, India, and China. This oil is used in making soaps, candles, burning oil, Russian varnishes, and Dutch enamel paint. The stems and leaves are used as fodder for cattle while the flowers are a source of honey. Finally, the pith from the stems is employed as a mounting medium in preparing microscope slides.

Sunflower leaves have long been employed as a home remedy in the Caucasus for malarial fevers. Several papers which appear in the medical literature recommend the use of the flowers in treating various illnesses, including the dilation of a bronchus or for fevers.

The leaves have even been dried and used as a substitute for tobacco in cigars. The flavor is said to resemble that of mild Spanish tobacco.

BOILS

✑ YELLOW DOCK

To bring about a discharge of pus, the Teton Dakota tribe tied several crushed yellow dock leaves to boils. The Ojibwas applied the pulverized root to cuts, while related species were employed for a wide variety of complaints by the Choctaws, Chickasaws, Pimas, Wichitas, Pawnees, Houmas, and Meskwakis. Obviously, this genus was a popular plant in Indian medicine.

This imported European weed had been used in medicine from ancient times and was adopted by the American Indians after being introduced to this continent. Originally the root had been used as a laxative and as a mild astringent tonic. By the late 1800s, a decoction of the root in boiling water was found "useful in dyspepsia, gouty tendencies, hepatic congestion, scrofula, syphilis, leprosy, elephantiasis, and various forms of scabby eruptions . . . (and) is also considered an excellent dentifrice, especially where the gums are spongy." This lengthy list of medical uses is not included to make our great grandfather's physicians appear gullible. Rather, I conclude that when a remedy proved valuable in the treatment of any one complaint, it was then tried on many other illnesses, and probably worked in some cases. This might be called the empirical method of healing—try everything and something is bound to work!

By the time the twentieth century rolled around, the roots of the same plant were recognized in official American medical circles and were recommended "for purifying the blood and in the treatment of skin diseases."

Even though the roots of yellow dock were accepted in the U.S. *Pharmacopoeia* from 1863 to 1905, a later writer stated in the *Dispensatory of the United States*, "Dock root is mildly laxative and astringent and in the days of legendary therapeutics was employed in syphilis and chronic skin diseases, but has no real value." What might a future medical writer say about certain of our present "scientific" pharmaceuticals?

✑ HORNED EUPHORBIA

The Navajos named the horned euphorbia, a member of the spurge family, pimple medicine. The plant was chewed and applied as a liniment for boils and pimples.

✑ WILD PANSY

In the seventeeth century, it was reported that an unidentified Indian tribe commonly utilized the crushed leaves of a yellow-flowered pansy on boils and swellings. However, the use of the pansy in medicine can be traced far back to ancient herbalists. Therefore, the Indians may have borrowed this plant remedy from the newly arrived Europeans.

By the late 1800s, the wild pansy was being ground up and used for various skin diseases, including impetigo, skin ulcers, and scabies.

This beautiful little species has become naturalized in this country and grows wild in dry, sandy soils, blossoming from April until July. The genus is widely cultivated, and numerous varieties have been encouraged.

Other plants utilized for boils by the Indians include blue flax, which was favored by the Paiute and Shoshoni tribes; the common selfheal, a remedy of the Quileute Indians of Washington; corn, which was employed as a poultice for boils, burns, and inflammations by the early settlers who may have improvised from an Indian remedy; Virginia anemone, the root of which was pulverized and applied as a wet poultice by the Menominees; and the glacier lily, which was a favorite boil medicine of the Blackfoot Indians. The root of this last-named species was also pulverized and applied as a wet dressing on skin sores.

As a standby remedy, the Indians always relied upon one of our most useful group of trees, the pines. The Choctaws of Louisiana treated boils and skin sores with a salve composed of pine gum, wax, and animal fat. Pine gum was also commonly rubbed on cuts and wounds with many successes reported. A favorite Indian gunshot treatment consisted of applying the inner bark of pine after it had first been soaked in water and softened.

BRONCHITIS

❧ WILD BERGAMOT

The Flambeau Ojibwa tribe boiled the dried wild bergamot and extracted bergamot oil which was inhaled to relieve bronchial complaints. The plant was also employed for colds by the Menominee, Meskwaki, and the Koasati tribes. Surprisingly, very little research has been done on this very active species. The chemists have extracted thymol from the leaves and flowering tops, and physicians have prescribed this volatile oil as a stimulant and to remove gases from the digestive tract. It is surprising that the Indian applications of this native plant for colds and bronchitis have not received wide attention.

Wild bergamot grows on dry hills and in thickets from Maine to Ontario and Minnesota and south to Florida, Louisiana, and Kansas. It has a slender stem, usually branched, two to three feet high. The leaves are thin and oval-lance-shaped, about one to four inches long. The flowers are lilac to pinkish in color and bear a hairy tuft on the upper lip. The stamens grow outside of the flower. The leaves were boiled and eaten with meat by the Tewa Indians, and a hair pomade of the boiled plant was employed by the Omaha and Ponca Indians.

❧ CREOSOTE BUSH

Although the creosote bush was used frequently and in many ways by Indian tribes of the Southwest, a tea of the leaves was employed for bronchial and other respiratory problems only by American practitioners. Creosote was official in the *U.S. Pharmacopoeia* from 1842 through 1942 and was used as an expectorant and pulmonary antiseptic.

❧ BALSAM POPLAR

The Pillager Ojibwas sought out the leaf buds of the balsam poplar for its resinous exudate, which has an invigorating balsamic odor. They made a salve of these buds mixed with bear or mutton fat and pressed the ointment into the nose to inhale the stimulating odor of balsam for relief of congestion due to colds and bronchitis.

Poplar buds were official in the *National Formulary* from 1916 to 1965 when they were employed like the turpentines. They are now little used in medicine but are recognized as an expectorant in subacute or chronic bronchitis. This is a fine example of an Indian remedy that has proved valuable for hundreds of years and is still valued today.

The tacamahac, or balsam poplar, grows about eighty feet high, has smooth gray bark, and a trunk diameter of seven feet. The leaves are broadly oval, three to five inches in length, and are dark green and shining on top and pale green below. The tree is especially abundant along streams and lakes from Newfoundland to Alaska and in the northern United States. The resinous buds, which resist freezing, flow with their fragrant "sap" throughout winter. The soft wood is sometimes used in the manufacture of boxes and is also wasted as paper pulp and excelsior.

❧ PLEURISY ROOT (FIG. 21)

The varieties of respiratory ailments treated with the pleurisy root species were by no means limited to the illness described by its common name. Not only was the species utilized as a remedy for pleurisy, but consumption, rheumatism, and bronchitis were also thought to be relieved by chewing the dried root. As for Indian usage, the Natchez drank a tea of the boiled roots as a remedy for pneumonia, while the Catawbas employed the same preparation for dysentery. The Omaha Indians chewed the fresh root for bronchitis and other respiratory complaints.

In the latter years of the nineteenth century, this native plant received a great deal of attention in medical circles and was much used as an expectorant, i.e., an agent used to promote the

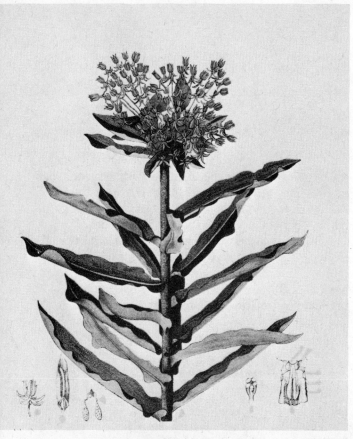

(FIG. 21) PLEURISY ROOT: *The Omaha Indians chewed the fresh root to treat bronchitis and other respiratory complaints. In the late nineteenth century this attractive plant was widely used as an expectorant in domestic American medicine.*

expulsion of phlegm. Dr. Millspaugh related the words of a colleague (1887):

> From the successful employment of the pleurisy-root for twenty-five years, he has imbibed such confidence that he extols it as possessing the peculiar and almost specific quality of acting on the organs of respiration, powerfully promoting suppressed expectoration, and thereby relieving the breathing of pleuritic patients in the most advanced stage of the disease; and in pneumonic fevers, recent colds, catarrhs, and diseases of the breast in general, this remedy has in his hands proved equally efficacious.

Even though several physicians of that time doubted its effectiveness, Millspaugh quoted another colleague who concluded that "from all that can be gathered on the subject, it may be deemed one of the most useful of our native articles, and deserves a full and unbiased trial."

The plant may have been given that trial and found useful, for in 1909, the root was selling for six to ten cents a pound wholesale. It was then being used "to promote expectoration, relieve pains in the chest, and induce easier breathing." Although the pleurisy root was continuously entered in the U.S. *Pharmacopoeia* from 1820 to 1905 and in the *National Formulary* from 1916 to 1936, the plant seems not yet to have had a fair trial in the laboratory and would appear to be a good candidate for renewed research. Maybe the Indians who preceded us on this continent had a valuable cure which we borrowed but never really examined?

This attractive plant flourishes in the open, in dry sandy soil, along roadsides or stream banks. It ranges from southeastern Canada to Florida, Texas, and Arizona. The erect stem grows about one to two feet in length and bears a thick growth of leaves. It bears conspicuous large umbels of brilliant, orange-colored flowers, usually from June to September. The flowers are followed by seed pods from four to five inches long that are edible and were boiled with buffalo meat by the western Indians. This is the only member of the genus that does not have the milky juice common to the milkweed family. It must be remembered that many members of this family are poisonous and that the raw, uncooked roots may be dangerous to eat.

WORMWOOD (FIG. 22)

The Yokia Indians of Mendocino County used a tea of the boiled leaves of an indigenous species of wormwood to cure bronchitis. Although it was not frequently employed in medicines, another indigenous species (*A. frigida*) is used as a source of camphor. Other native species have been utilized by several tribes for diverse purposes.

The Kiowa, a Plains tribe, chewed the leaves of Mexican mugwort for sore throat, while leaves of the black sage were chewed by the Tewa Indians to expel gas from the intestinal tract.

The best-known plant of this genus is from Europe (*A. absinthium*). This species was formerly utilized to make the French drink absinthe before its sale was made illegal.

European wormwood had been used in medicine from ancient times. In the time of Dioscorides and Pliny, it was used against worms for which use it has inherited its common name. Through the ages it has been employed for treating a wide variety of ailments, including scurvy, gout, and epilepsy. The volatile oil, however, has been proved to be an active, narcotic poison and is no longer used.

The stimulating drink absinthe was compounded from green anise, star anise, large absinthe, small absinthe, coriander, and hyssop. These were distilled together until the distillate became reddish, and then the following herbs were added for color and flavor: peppermint, balm, lemon peel, and licorice root.

This must have been a very good drink because it claimed many "absintheics" whose habit is described in the *Dispensatory of the United States*: "restlessness at night, with disturbing dreams, nausea and vomiting in the morning, with great trembling of the hands and tongue, vertigo, and a tendency to epileptiform convulsions."

But perhaps the drink was made illegal because of incidents similar to the case described by Dr. Millspaugh in 1887:

A druggist's clerk took about half an ounce of the oil; he was found on the floor perfectly insensible, convulsed, and foaming at the mouth; shortly afterward the convulsions ceased, the patient remained insensible with the jaws locked, pupils dilated, pulse weak, and stomach retching . . . the man recovered but could not remember how or when he had taken the drug . . . Dr. Magnan, who had a great number of absinthe drinkers under his care . . . states that peculiar epileptic attacks result, which he has called "absinthe epilepsy."

But this is a long way from American Indian plant remedies, so we shall now turn to their methods of treating burns.

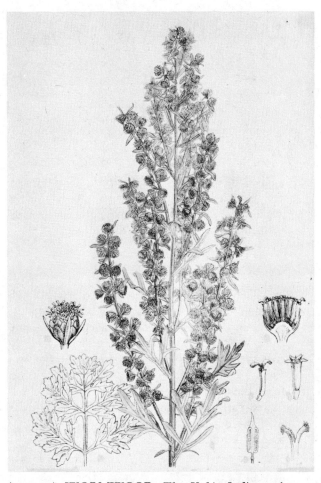

(FIG. 22) WORMWOOD: *The Yokia Indians of Mendocino County used a tea of the boiled leaves of a local species of wormwood to cure bronchitis. European wormwood (above) was formerly used to make absinthe.*

BURNS

❦ HORSETAIL FERNS

The Thompson tribe of British Columbia applied the ashes of horsetail fern stems to serious burns and then bandaged the wound with a clean cloth. Sometimes, animal fats were mixed with the ashes to prepare burn ointment.

❦ SCARLET MALLOW

The Blackfoot Indians chewed scarlet mallow and applied its mucilagenous paste to scalds, sores, and burns as a cooling agent. The same paste was sometimes used by medicine men to coat their arms and hands before reaching into a pan of boiling water. This protected their skin from the heat and enabled them to appear endowed with supernatural powers. The same tribe used the down of common cattail as a dressing, to pack burns.

❦ YELLOW-SPINED THISTLE

The Kiowa Indians boiled yellow-spined thistle blossoms and applied the resulting liquid to burns and skin sores. They considered this an excellent remedy and also utilized the roots of this plant as food. The Zuñi drank a tea of the entire plant boiled in water as a cure for syphilis, but little else is reported on the use of this thistle in medicines.

❦ YARROW

The showy yarrow plant was also very frequently used for wounds and is treated in greater detail under that category. For burns, the Zuñi Indians of New Mexico ground the entire plant, steeped it in cold water, and used the liquid to bring about a cooling sensation. Yarrow contains a dark blue volatile oil, cineol, which may explain its stimulating properties.

The Little Lake Indians of Mendocino County, California, applied the yellow, pitchy gum of the

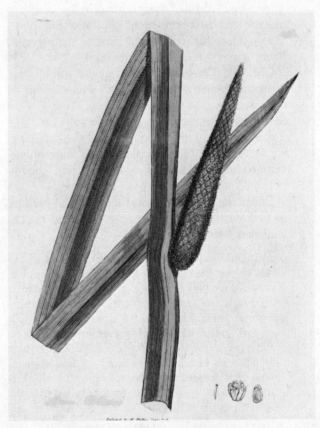

(FIG. 23) SWEET FLAG: *The Meskwakis applied the boiled root to burns.*

digger pine as a protective, healing covering for burns and sores. The resin of the balsam fir was employed for the same purposes by the Penobscots of Maine while the Meskwakis used the boiled root of sweet flag (FIG. 23). Forest Indians boiled the inner bark of basswood and applied the liquid to soothe and soften the burned skin. A report to the American Medical Association in 1849 praised this remedy for its effectiveness.

The Navajo Indians used several different plants for burns. Among these are four-o'clock, hairy umbrella wort, penstemon, and sagebrush. These plants were prepared individually as dusting powders, lotions, and poultices. Ointments were prepared by pulverizing the plant together with sheep fat and red ochre.

CENTIPEDE BITES

‌ PAINTED CUP

The blossoms of painted cup and the blossoms of penstemon were steeped together in hot water, and the resulting liquid was applied to painful centipede bites by the Navajo Indians. This plant may have been used on these painful, burning wounds because the red, flamelike flowers hinted to the Navajo and other Indians of its properties according to the "doctrine of signatures," the ancient medical theory which held that the usefulness of a plant could be determined by its shape, color, odor, etc. Thus, if a plant had heart-shaped leaves, it was good for heart troubles, or if the plant blazed at you in its colors, it would be good on burns.

Leslie Haskin, a Pacific Coast botanist, relates an interesting tale of the Chinook Indians which corroborates this theory:

Once when Bluejay (a tribal god) was about to go upon a journey he was given five buckets full of water with which to quench five burning prairies through which he would have to pass. Coming, as he journeyed, to a meadow where red, flamelike flowers grew—the weather being exceedingly hot—he was deceived into thinking that this was the fire of which he had been warned, and in an attempt to quench the blazing flowers, poured out and wasted a great deal of the water. Later, coming to the real fires, he had not enough left, and in attempting to pass he perished. (from *Wild Flowers of the Pacific Coast* by L. Haskin, 1967)

Only one other remedy for centipede bites appears in the literature. This is Venus's-hair. The Kayenta Navajo steeped that portion of the fern which grows above ground in hot water and applied the liquid as a rinse. The same solution was also used for bumblebee stings.

CHILDBIRTH

For purposes of organization this childbirth section will be treated in the following four categories: (1) to speed childbirth; (2) to speed delivery of the placenta; (3) to stop post-partem hemorrhage; (4) to relieve the pain.

1. TO SPEED CHILDBIRTH:

✑ PARTRIDGEBERRY (FIG.24)

As is common in the case of plants employed for "female troubles," the Indians were reluctant to deliver much information about their methods of preparation and specific applications for the partridgeberry, also called squaw vine. The Cherokees told one investigator that they used a tea of the leaves boiled in water. This same preparation was later confirmed among the Penobscots of Maine. Frequent doses of the tea were taken in the few weeks preceding the expected date of delivery.

This plant soon became very popular as a home treatment to speed labor and was admitted into the *National Formulary* in 1926 where it remained until 1947. The leaves were used for their tonic, astringent, and diuretic properties.

This beautiful, little evergreen herb is found creeping about in the moss at the foot of forest trees and decayed stumps. It grows between six and fourteen inches in height and shows thick, shining, dark green opposite leaves about half an inch in length. The leaves sometimes show whitish veins. Fragrant white flowers, which are funnel-shaped, appear from about April to June. The scarlet fruits are very prominent and remain on the vine through the winter. These are edible though practically devoid of taste.

✑ BLUE COHOSH (FIG.25)

The native blue cohosh was widely used as an aid to parturition, first by the Indians and then by the early white settlers who called it squawroot and papoose root. To promote a rapid delivery, an infusion of the root in warm water was drunk as a tea for a week or two prior to the expected date of delivery. This same preparation was taken by various tribes for other purposes as well. The Menominees, Ojibwas,

(FIG. 24) PARTRIDGEBERRY: *A tea made of the leaves was taken by Cherokee women to speed labor.*

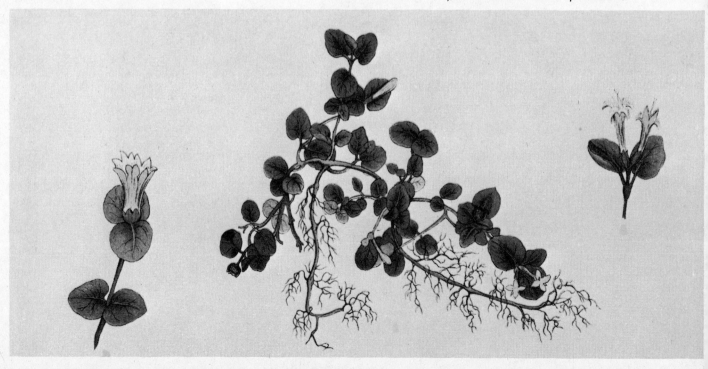

Meskwakis, and Potawatomis used it for "female troubles," while among the Omahas, a boiled decoction of the root was a favorite remedy for fever.

Around 1909, blue cohosh root was actively being collected and traded and was bringing a wholesale price of from two and one-half to four cents a pound. The dried root was official in the *U.S. Pharmacopoeia* from 1882 to 1905 when it

less leaf appears at the top and divides into three stems which again divide into threes. Blue cohosh, which attains a height of from one to three feet, bears small, greenish flowers from April to May and round bluish seeds around August which resemble berries. The seeds are said to be an excellent substitute for coffee when roasted. When used medicinally, the roots are collected in the fall when they are richest in their chemical constituents.

Another plant which was employed to speed childbirth is the balsam fir. The Ottawa, Chippewa, and Tewa Indians all prepared the inner bark of this tree in boiling water, mixed in tobacco leaves, and inhaled the rising steam. In this case, the balsamic odor probably stimulated the squaw's nasal passages but did little else. For the same purpose and probably yielding the same nil effect, Ottawa and Chippewa women drank a tea of the inner bark of the yellow pine.

2. TO SPEED DELIVERY OF THE PLACENTA:

AMERICAN LICORICE

The edible roots of the American licorice were boiled in water and the resulting tea drunk by the early white settlers who either learned to use this plant from the Indians or adapted an earlier European remedy from the common licorice of Europe. This latter species is used medicinally as a laxative, to promote the expulsion of phlegm, and for masking the taste of bitter drugs. The roots of both species are edible, and American licorice was sometimes cultivated by the Indians.

BROOM SNAKEWEED

Navajo women drank a tea of the whole broom snakeweed to promote the expulsion of the placenta. This resinous plant was also chewed and then applied to bee, ant, and wasp stings by the same tribe. The Hopi Indians sometimes employed snakeweed tea for gastric upsets. This perennial is abundant in northern Arizona and shows yellow ray flowers from July through October.

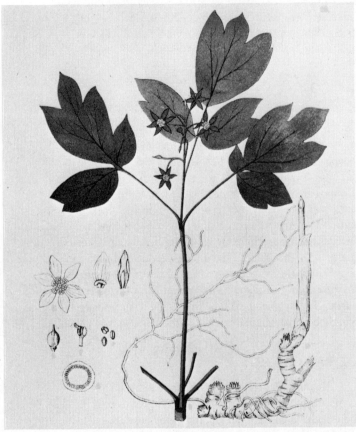

(FIG. 25) BLUE COHOSH: *This native plant was widely used to speed childbirth first by the Indians and then by the early white settlers who named it squawroot.*

was used for antispasmodic, emmenagogue, and diuretic purposes. One clinician found that an extract of the root has a pronounced stimulating effect on the uterine muscle.

This perennial herb shuns the open fields and busy roadsides, remaining hidden in the deep recesses of shady woods from New Brunswick to South Carolina and west to Nebraska. It grows most abundantly throughout the Allegheny Mountain region. As illustrated, the large, almost stem-

3. TO STOP POST-PARTEM HEMORRHAGE:

ᴥ§ BUCKWHEAT

Hopi women were given an infusion of the entire buckwheat plant to stop post-partem bleeding.

ᴥ§ BLACK WESTERN CHOKECHERRY

Arikara women were given a drink of the berry juice of black western chokecherries to stop bleeding following delivery. For the same purpose they sometimes drank a tea of the pulverized root of mallow mixed with the gummy exudate of the chokecherry tree.

ᴥ§ JUNIPER

Although not used to stop bleeding, a tea of juniper leaves was drunk by Zuñi women to relax their muscles following delivery. Juniper berries are eaten by birds, bears, and other wildlife and are sometimes eaten in emergencies by man. The berries of the common juniper are used in the making of gin to provide the flavor.

ᴥ§ SMOOTH UPLAND SUMAC

The Omahas boiled the smooth upland sumac fruits and applied the liquid as an external wash to stop bleeding following delivery.

4. TO RELIEVE THE PAIN OF CHILDBIRTH:

ᴥ§ WILD BLACK CHERRY

The black cherry plant has well-documented calming properties and is treated in greater detail under "Sedatives." Cherokee women were given a tea of the inner bark to relieve pain in the early stages of labor. This preparation was soon adopted by the early settlers and became official in the U.S. *Pharmacopoeia* in 1820 where the bark is still listed for its sedative properties.

ᴥ§ COTTON

The Alabama and Koasati tribes made a tea of the roots of the very useful cotton plant to relieve the pains of labor. Cotton was listed for its abortifacient properties in the U.S. *Pharmacopoeia* from 1863 to 1950. Cotton has been known since ancient times. More than four thousand years ago Egypt had an important cotton industry, and the plant has been cultivated in India for more than three thousand years. Remains of the plant have been found in the mounds of the Mexican Aztecs, which are thought to antedate the Egyptian pyramids. The genus name, *Gossypium*, comes from the Arabic *goz* which describes a "soft silky substance."

ᴥ§ LADY FERN

To relieve labor pains, the Washington Indians employed a tea of the boiled stems of the lady fern. General body pains were treated with a tea of the boiled rhizomes of this fern.

COLDS

A cold may be described by its symptoms, and many remedies have been used for coughs, running noses, lack of energy, etc. In the following list I describe remedies that were used to treat these symptoms when they occurred simultaneously. For specific complaints, such as cough, check each category in the table of contents.

✑ BONESET (FIG.26)

"There is probably no plant in American domestic practice that has more extensive or frequent use than this [boneset]." So wrote Dr. C. F. Millspaugh in 1887, and he continued to extol the powers of this common weed.

> The attic, or woodshed, of almost every country farm-house, has its bunches of the dried herb hanging tops downward from the rafters during the whole year, ready for immediate use should some member of the family, or that of a neighbor, be taken with a cold. How many children have winched when the maternal edit: "drink this boneset; it'll do you good" has been issued; and how many old men have craned their necks to allow the nauseous draught to the quicker pass the palate! The use of a hot infusion of the tops and leaves to produce diaphoresis [profuse sweating] was handed down to the early settlers of this country by the Aborigines. . . .

And Indian usage of boneset was widespread. The Menominees used it to reduce fever; the Alabamas, to relieve stomachache; the Creeks, for body pain; the Iroquois and the Mohegans, for fever and colds.

Dr. Millspaugh continues, with a description of his friend, a physician, who suffered from intermittent fever (probably malarial):

> When he was a young man, living in the central part of this State, he was attacked with intermittent fever, which lasted off and on for three years. Being of a bilious temperament, he grew at length sallow, emaciated, and hardly able to get about. As he sat one day, resting by the side of the road, an old lady of his acquaintance told him to go

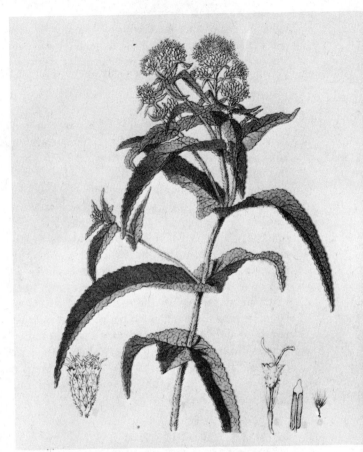

(FIG. 26) BONESET: *Boneset tea was one of the most frequently used home remedies during the last century. It was borrowed from the Indians who had used it to reduce fever, to relieve body pains, and to treat colds.*

home and have some boneset "fixed," and it would certainly cure him. (He had been given, during the years he suffered, quinine, cinchonine bark and all its known derivatives, as well as cholagogues, and every other substance then known to the regular practitioner, without effect; the attacks coming on latterly twice a day.) On reaching home, with the aid of the fences and buildings along the way, he received a tablespoonful of a decoction of boneset evaporated until it was about the consistency of syrup, and immediately went to bed. He had hardly lain down when insensibility and stupor came on, passing into deep sleep. On awakening in the morning, he felt decidedly better, and from that moment improved rapidly without farther medication, gaining flesh and strength daily. No attack returned for twenty years, when a short one was brought on by lying down in a marsh while hunting.

Boneset was a favorite remedy for fever and colds at least one hundred years before it was listed in any American medical text. It was introduced to England for its medical properties in 1699, and by the time Dr. Millspaugh's book was published in 1887, boneset was listed in every book treating North American medical botany. The dried leaves and flowering tops were entered in the *U.S. Pharmacopoeia* from 1820 through 1916 and in the *National Formulary* from 1926 through 1950.

Boneset is commonly found in wet ground, along streams and near swamps and thickets from Canada to Florida and west to Texas and Nebraska. As illustrated, this weed has leaves which are opposite each other, but which are united at their bases. This unique arrangement makes it appear as though the two leaves were only one, with the stem passing through the center. This hairy-stemmed boneset grows between one and five feet high and bears clusters of small white tubular flowers from about July to September. When to be used in medicines, the leaves and flowering tops were collected during August, or when the plant was in flower.

✑ BALM OF GILEAD BUDS

Balm of Gilead buds are derived from a certain type of poplar tree. These buds are covered with a resinous sap which has a strong turpentinelike odor and a bitter taste. The Menominee Indians prepared an inhalant from these buds boiled in animal fat. To relieve congested nasal passages, this ointment was inhaled, the turpentinelike odor of the balsam stimulating and invigorating the tissues of the respiratory passages.

These buds are rich in salicin, a glucoside that probably decomposes into salicylic acid in the human system. Since aspirin is made by combining salicylic acid and acetic anhydride, the effects of salicin, from balm of Gilead buds, may be similar to those of aspirin in some respects. This is another example of empirical reasoning.

The Indian who searched the forests for his cures tried several plants going only on scant mythological leads. If he stumbled on a poisonous plant and unknowingly chewed its root, perhaps that was the end of a budding practitioner. If, however, he avoided the poisonous species, chewed another plant, and found himself feeling better, he probably described the curing effects in his tales, and the plant became accepted in the tribal plant armamentorium. So with the balm of Gilead buds; when the balsam was inhaled, the Indian who was suffering from stuffed respiratory passages due to a cold was relieved, and these little leaf buds became an accepted Indian remedy.

These buds were official in the *National Formulary* from 1916 to 1965 when they were used to promote the expulsion of phlegm and for their stimulant properties.

The large member of the willow family, which produces these buds, sometimes grows as high as one hundred feet with a trunk as broad as six and one-half feet in diameter. The generic name, *Populus*, refers to the Latin name of the poplar (*arbor populi*) meaning "the people's tree," so called because it was widely planted on boulevards. The balm of Gilead tree has broad, ovate leaves between two and one-half and six inches long which are narrowed at the base and pointed at the apex. They are dark green above and pale green on the lower surface. The tree is found along streams and roadsides from Newfoundland to Virginia and north to Michigan, South Dakota, and Alaska.

✑ WINTERGREEN (FIG. 27)

Although the name wintergreen has been ascribed to many genera of plants, notably *Pyrola*, *Chimaphila*, *Moneses*, and *Gaultheria*, the species herein described and illustrated (*Gaultheria*) was the most popular in domestic American medicine. Also known as checkerberry, wintergreen was utilized in Indian medicine and is described by Thoreau who imbibed the leaves as a tea prepared by his Indian guide.

The leaves yield an oil on steam distillation that is a valuable flavoring agent and is also considered antirheumatic. Oil of wintergreen, or methyl salicylate, was formerly used as a folk remedy for body aches and pains. A piece of cloth was soaked in the aromatic liquid and then tied

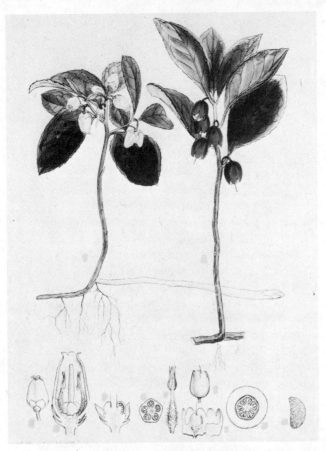

(FIG. 27) WINTERGREEN: *Oil of wintergreen was formerly used as a folk remedy for body aches and pains. It has been used in Indian medicine and is described by Thoreau, who drank a tea made of the leaves as prepared by his Indian guide.*

to offending joints. Methyl salicylate is closely related to acetylsalicylic acid, or aspirin. Wintergreen leaves were official in the *U.S. Pharmacopoeia* from 1820 to 1894, while the oil of wintergreen is still listed for its astringent, diuretic, and stimulant properties.

The bright red berries and the young leaves of this small native perennial are edible, being the principal food of partridges, grouse, and deer in the late fall. The plant occurs in cool, damp forests, especially beneath evergreen trees in Canada and the northeastern United States. It seldom exceeds six inches in height, bears alternate leaves which are shining, dark green above, and thick and leathery to the touch. The white, waxy flowers appear from about June to September; these are followed by bright red berries which ripen in the fall and remain on the plant through the winter months. The plant has a characteristic oil of wintergreen smell and taste. When used in medicines, the leaves are collected in autumn and dried.

ᛞᴈ WORMWOOD

In addition to the information already given for the wormwood plants under "Bronchitis," it is known that the Zuñi Indians of western New Mexico utilized a tea of the leaves for colds and that the Thompson Indians of British Columbia drank a decoction of the boiled stems, leaves, and twigs of a species of wormwood, black sage, for the same affliction. The crushed leaves of this plant emit a powerful odor—the Thompsons sometimes stuffed the nostrils with them to relieve nasal congestion. They were also employed by this tribe when the men were required to bury decaying corpses. By stuffing the leaves into their nostrils, the burial party avoided one aspect of an unpleasant situation.

Artemisia frigida, a species of wormwood, contains camphor; this substance is still listed in the *U.S. Pharmacopoeia* where it is described as a stimulant and antispasmodic agent.

The following plants are either treated elsewhere in this book or are not sufficiently well-known Indian cold remedies to warrant extensive coverage.

The Cherokees steeped the leaves of the chinquapin tree and employed the liquid as an external wash for the feverish conditions common to colds.

The Navajos drank a tea of wild bergamot to reduce low fevers and to soothe sore throat, headache, and colds. The same tribe sometimes chewed the root of black root for coughs and colds or bathed the patient in a bath of bigelow sagebrush. The Hopi Indians treated colds with a tea of wild rhubarb while the Forest Potawatomi tribe made a root tea of the black-eyed Susan. Some tribes chewed sweet flag roots and drank a decoction for colds, while the Potawatomis inhaled small grains of the pulverized root to stop running noses. The Pillager Ojibwas used a tea of this species for throat colds. Finally, we again come upon another useful pine tree, the white pine. The Mohegans steeped the inner bark of it in warm water and drank the tea to cure colds.

One of the most universally used items of the Indians was the sweat bath. It was utilized for treating every ailment, especially valued in treating colds, respiratory ailments, and rheumatism. A detailed description of several Indian sweat lodges appears under "Rheumatism."

COLIC

ᴥ CATNIP (FIG.28)

The Mohegans made a tea of catnip leaves for infantile colic. This became a popular domestic remedy and is still used today in some regions of the United States. Catnip is also used to induce sweating to cure colds. At the beginning of this century, the leaves and flowering tops were widely used in medicine as a stimulant or to promote suppressed menstruation. The plant was also thought to have a sedative effect. It was official in the *U.S. Pharmacopoeia* from 1842 through

(FIG. 28) *CATNIP: The Mohegans used a tea made of the leaves to relieve infantile colic. This became a popular remedy among the early settlers and is still used today in some regions of the United States.*

1882 and in the *National Formulary* from 1916 to 1950. Man popularly thinks that cats are attracted to it because it acts as a feline aphrodisiac.

This introduced weed occurs in dry soil from Canada to Minnesota and south to Virginia and Arkansas. It grows to a height of about two to three feet and bears heart-shaped, scalloped leaves that are green above and grayish green below. The whitish flowers grow in dense spikes at the ends of stems and branches from June to September. When used medicinally, the leaves and flowering tops were collected when the plant was in flower and then dried.

ᴥ AMERICAN ELDER (FIG.29)

The Mohegans prepared a tea of the flowers of the small American elder shrub for babies discomforted by colic. It is difficult to appraise the

(FIG. 29) *AMERICAN ELDER: The Mohegans prepared a tea from the flowers of this small shrub for babies discomforted by colic.*

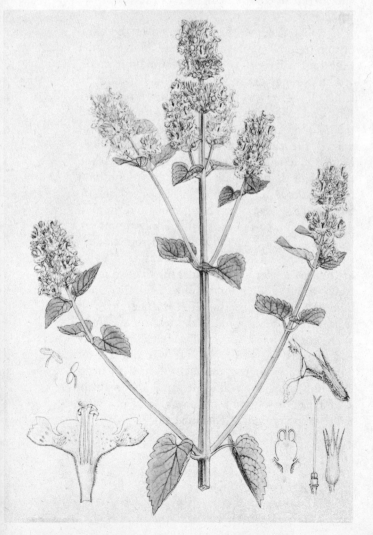

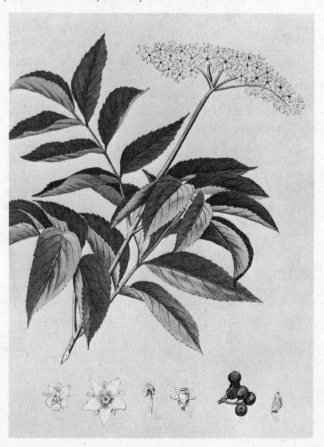

value of such a remedy because colic is so vague a disorder; however, the plant was employed by several other tribes for different purposes. The Menominees drank a tea of the dried flowers to reduce fevers, while the Houma Indians prepared a wash of the boiled bark for inflammations. The Meskwakis used a tea of the root bark to encourage the expulsion of phlegm, to treat headache, and to encourage labor.

Probably because of this wide Indian usage, elder became an important ingredient in the home remedies of many whites. To treat wounds a wash of the boiled flowers or leaves was applied; a tea of the flowers was employed in colds to induce sweating; the berries were utilized to make a cooling, laxative drink.

Elderberries were entered in the *U.S. Pharmacopoeia* from 1820 to 1831 when their juice was used for wine. Elder flowers were in the *U.S. Pharmacopoeia* from 1831 to 1905 when they were used to make a flower water and as a flavoring. One text on pharmacognosy lists the properties of elder flowers as stimulant, diuretic, and sweat inducing.

This branching shrub grows in low, moist grounds from Nova Scotia to Florida and west to Manitoba, Kansas, and Texas. Its trunk is covered with a yellowish gray bark, and the small white flowers appear from May to July. The dark purple fruits, which appear in early autumn, are commonly used as preservatives or to prepare a wine.

CONTRACEPTIVES

The motivations for avoiding pregnancy are probably the same as those assembled by Devereux regarding voluntary abortion. Harold E. Driver evaluated Devereux's data for ninety North American Indian cultures and generalized the motivations for abortion as follows:

> . . . illegitimacy of the pregnancy; desire to avoid the trouble and work of rearing children; fear of the pain, of injury to the mother's health, or of death at childbirth; poverty of the parents; desire to avoid bringing a child into the modern world with its discrimination against Indians and half-breeds; quarrels between parents and desertion of a pregnant woman by her husband or lover; fear of bringing into the world a child associated with coitus taboos, such as those during pregnancy or during the nursing period of a previous child; desire to avoid producing a child who will become a slave, a prisoner of war, or a person of any other undesirable status; desire to avoid producing offspring from an adulterous union. (From *Indians of North America*, by H. E. Driver, p. 434)

Following are some of the plants used to prevent pregnancy.

RAGLEAF BAHIA

The Navajos, who called the ragleaf bahia herb twisted medicine, drank a tea of the roots boiled in water for thirty minutes for contraceptive purposes. They also used this plant as an arthritis medicine. It is found inside of the Grand Canyon and on both rims, and flowers from July to November in the Tusayan Ruins area of the park.

INDIAN PAINTBRUSH

Hopi women drank a tea of the whole Indian paintbrush to "dry up the menstrual flow."

BLUE COHOSH

Chippewa women drank a strong decoction of the powdered blue cohosh root to promote parturition and menstruation.

DOGBANE

The dogbane plant, which was most frequently used by the Indians to rid the body of excess fluids, was regarded by them as a "kidney or heart" medicine. Dogbane is included in a list of "Plant Materials Used by Primitive Peoples to Affect Fertility," which was compiled by DeLaszlo and Henshaw. Without naming the Indian tribe, these scientists wrote that dogbane was employed in North America as a contraceptive. The preparation consisted of the roots boiled in water and was drunk once weekly.

WILD GINGER

The root and rhizome of wild ginger were boiled slowly in a small quantity of water for a long period of time, and the resulting decoction drunk by women of an undesignated tribe of North American Indians.

WATER HEMLOCK (FIG.30)

Cherokee women chewed and swallowed water hemlock root for four consecutive days to induce permanent sterility. Rafinesque, an eighteenth-century botanist, claimed that "its roots were eaten by such Indians as were tired of life and desired a speedy demise." The plant is highly poisonous, and many deaths following ingestion have been reported. The poisonous principle of cowbane, called cicutoxin, is related to picrotoxin, a powerful stimulant of the central nervous system. Another common name for this poisonous

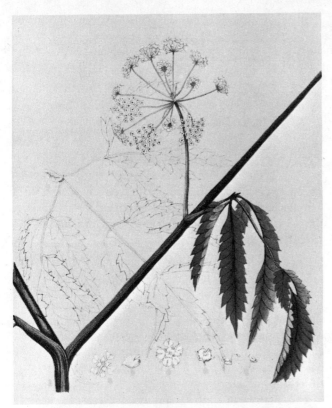

(FIG. 30) WATER HEMLOCK: *Cherokee women chewed and swallowed the root of this highly poisonous marsh dweller to induce permanent sterility.*

marsh perennial is death of man; Dr. C. F. Millspaugh describes one of its victims:

A boy had eaten of certain tuberous roots, gathered in a recently-ploughed field, supposing them to be artichokes, but which were identified as the roots of *Cicuta maculata*. His first symptom was a pain in the bowels urging him to an ineffectual attempt at stool, after which he vomited about a teacupful of what appeared to be the recently masticated root, and immediately fell back into convulsions which lasted off and on continuously until his death.

❧ MILKWEED

Navajo women drank a tea prepared of the whole milkweed plant after childbirth. To promote temporary sterility, Indians of Quebec, Canada, drank an infusion of the pounded roots of a related species of milkweed (*A. syriaca*).

❧ AMERICAN MISTLETOE

The Indians of Mendocino County, California, drank a tea of the American mistletoe leaves to induce abortion or to prevent conception.

❧ ANTELOPE SAGE

To prevent conception, Navajo women drank one cup of a decoction of boiled antelope sage root during menstruation. The Zuñi Indians used the root to cure many illnesses.

❧ FALSE SOLOMON'S-SEAL

The Nevada Indians drank a root tea prepared from false Solomon's-seal to regulate menstrual disorders, and prevented conception by drinking one-half cup of a leaf tea daily for one week.

❧ STONESEED

Shoshoni women of Nevada reportedly drank a cold water infusion of stoneseed roots everyday for six months to ensure permanent sterility. Virgil J. Vogel reports that an experiment with mice, performed by Clellan Ford, has shown that alcoholic extracts of this plant eliminated the estrous cycle and decreased the weights of the ovaries, thymus, and pituitary glands. The scientist was so impressed with the activity of stoneseed in mice that he suggested that "the unit of activity in *Lithosperma* be expressed in terms of P.P.U.'s, i.e., Papoose Preventative Units."

The Shoshoni also occasionally drank an infusion of deer's-tongue as a contraceptive.

❧ THISTLE

The Quinault Indians of Washington steeped the whole thistle plant and drank the resulting tea to inhibit fertilization.

❧ INDIAN TURNIP

The Hopis used the native Indian turnip, or jack-in-the-pulpit, to induce temporary or permanent sterility, depending upon the dosage. It was believed that one teaspoonful of the powdered, dried root in one-half glass of cold water that was strained would prevent conception for one week, and that two teaspoonfuls of a hot infusion would render the individual permanently sterile.

COUGHS

∙§ ASPEN (FIG. 31)

The Cree Indians ate the inner bark of the beautiful white-trunked forest aspen for food; they also considered an infusion of it an excellent remedy for coughs.

Aspen bark, like willow bark, contains salicin which is thought to decompose into an aspirin-like compound in the human system, salicyclic acid. Although this was not known by our grand-

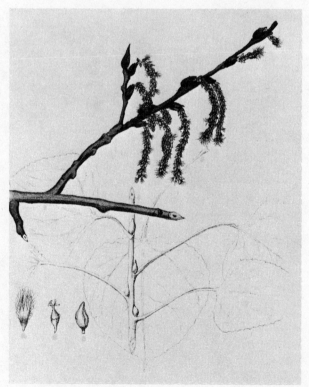

(FIG. 31) ASPEN: *The Cree Indians prepared a tea from the inner bark of this beautiful forest tree as a remedy for coughs.*

father's physicians, they seemed to rely upon aspen bark to treat fevers, to use in tonics, to promote sweating, and to act as a diuretic. Today, many physicians recommend aspirin for some of the above effects—it is interesting to see how some

of our present knowledge is derived from the "knowledge by doing" school of the doctors of the 1800s. The Indian, of course, was the most ardent student of experience.

∙§ WILD CHERRY

The bark of the wild cherry was at one time the most popular ingredient in home remedies for coughs and colds. Believed to exert a sedative effect on the nerves of respiration, the dried bark has been listed in the U.S. *Pharmacopoeia* continually since 1820.

The Flambeau Ojibwas prepared a tea of the bark of wild cherry for coughs and colds, while other tribes used a bark tea for diarrhea or for lung troubles. This plant is illustrated and described under "Sedatives."

∙§ WHITE PINE

The inner bark of the large evergreen white pine is still used as an ingredient in a commercial cough syrup. Several Indian tribes employed the bark for similar purposes in their native medicine. Usage of white pine is reported for most regions in which it is found where there was an indigenous people. The Ojibwas, Mohegans, Montagnais, Menominees, and Potawatomis all used parts of this tree in various ways: the bark as a tea for colds and coughs and the resinous exudate on sores and wounds or boiled in water for colds and respiratory ailments.

The dried inner bark contains up to 10 percent tannin, some mucilage, an oleoresin, a glycoside, and a volatile oil. As an ingredient in cough syrup, it is used for colds and coughs to promote the expulsion of phlegm from the respiratory passages. White pine bark was entered in the *National Formulary* from 1916 to 1965.

This large conifer sometimes grows up to two hundred feet high. It has a smooth, grayish green bark when young that becomes dark and rough as the tree ages. The pine needles of this species are about three to five inches long and usually five in a bunch. The cones are cylindrical and drooping, five to ten inches long, and sometimes curved. After the seeds fall out, in early autumn, the scales spread apart and the cones are much wider.

☙ SARSAPARILLA (FIG. 32)

Sarsaparilla was used extensively by the Indians and then borrowed by the whites. The Penobscots pulverized dried sarsaparilla roots and combined them with sweet flag roots in warm water, utilizing the dark liquid as a cough remedy. The Kwakiutl Indians of the northern Pacific coast region prepared a cough medicine from the pulverized root in an unspecified oil. Pillager Ojibwas affected with bad cough drank a decoction of the pulverized root boiled in water.

Sarsaparilla was once a popular drink in America; however, commercial varieties contained the roots of several other plants mixed with the roots of this plant. The Indians generally utilized sarsaparilla by itself. An early New England botanist reports that the Indians ate the roots during wars or hunts because they were able to subsist on them for long periods of time.

(FIG. 32) *JAMAICAN SARSAPARILLA: The roots were boiled in water by several tribes who used the resulting tea as a cough medicine.*

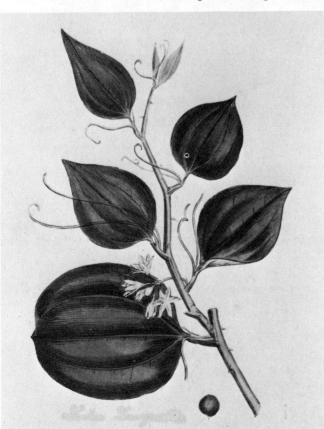

This plant, which belongs to the ginseng family, is very closely related, both botanically and chemically, to the spikenard, which is described and illustrated under "Backache." Both plants were used for their stimulant and sweat-inducing properties; sarsaparilla was official in the *U.S. Pharmacopoeia* from 1820 through 1882.

This native perennial has only one long-stalked leaf which is divided into three parts, each division bearing five oval, sharply toothed leaflets from two to five inches long. The naked flowering stalk usually bears three clusters of small, greenish white flowers from May to June. These are followed by round, purplish black berries. The dried rootstock, which is slightly aromatic, is collected in autumn. Wild sarsaparilla grows in moist woods from Newfoundland to Manitoba and south to North Carolina and Missouri.

☙ SENECA SNAKEROOT

Although the useful little Seneca snakeroot was widely employed by the Indians for treating the effects of snakebite (as implied by its name), it found acceptance in American and European medicine as an ingredient in a cough medicine. The history of this switch in usage is described by Dr. C. F. Millspaugh:

About the year 1735, John Tennent, a Scotch Physician, noted that the Seneca Indians obtained excellent effects from a certain plant, as a remedy for the bite of the rattlesnake; after considerable painstaking and much bribing, he was shown the roots and given to understand (they were) Seneca Snakeroot. Noting, then, that the symptoms of the bite were similar in some respects to that of pleurisy and the latter stages of peripneumonia, he conceived the idea of using this root also in those diseases. His success was such that he wrote to Dr. Mead, of London, the results of his experiments. His epistle was printed at Edinburgh in 1738, and the new drug favorably received throughout Europe, and cultivated in England in 1739.

Seneca snakeroot was claimed to be a stimulating expectorant and was used in pneumonia, asthma, and other respiratory ailments. The 23d edition of the *Dispensatory of the United States* notes that this plant has been used in bronchitis and asthma and that it owes its therapeutic value to the saponins contained within the dried root.

This work issues caution that in overdose, the plant is poisonous.

The following plants have received little attention as cough remedies but are listed for interest.

Indian tribes of the Missouri River region boiled the fruits and leaves of red cedar and utilized the dark drink for colds and coughs. The smoke from the smoldering leafy twigs was sometimes inhaled for head colds by the same tribes.

The Mohegans made what they considered to be "an excellent cough remedy" from mullein leaves steeped in molasses. The same tribe also steeped spikenard leaves in warm water or used the leaves of American chestnut in the same way to calm the respiratory nerves and to promote expectoration.

DANDRUFF

⋟ CORN

The oil of corn grains was rubbed into the scalp by the Chickasaws.

⋟ SWORD FERN

The Indians of California applied a decoction of boiled sword fern rhizome for dandruff while utilizing an infusion of the steeped fronds for boils and sores. Occasionally, the sporangia were dried and crushed and applied to burns.

⋟ ROCKY MOUNTAIN JUNIPER

The Hopi Indians rubbed the leaves of the bushy, shrublike Rocky Mountain juniper into their hair after bathing to remove dandruff.

⋟ SOAP ROOT

The roots of soap root were pounded and mixed with water by many tribes who used the "soapy" solution on their hair. The Kiowa considered this an effective treatment for dandruff and skin irritations.

⋟ WILLOW

An infusion of willow roots was used by the Chickasaws for treating nosebleeds, headache, and dysentery, while a solution of the leaves and young twigs was applied to an itchy scalp to remove dandruff.

DIABETES

✑ WILD CARROT (FIG.33)

Botanically, the wild carrot species is grouped closely to the devil's club. Whereas the last-named plant belongs to the ginseng family (as do spikenard and sarsaparilla), the wild carrot belongs to the ammiaceae, or carrot, family.

The Mohegans steeped the blossoms of this wild species in warm water when they were in full bloom and took the drink for diabetes. Crow Indians employed this plant for ceremonial purposes and also in undisclosed preparations for medicines.

Its beautiful flowers earned this plant the name Queen Anne's lace in Europe, its native environment. Carrot root had long been used in Europe as a remedy for threadworms, and the seeds were used for their diuretic properties. An excessive

(FIG. 33) WILD CARROT: *The Mohegans steeped the blossoms of this wild relative of our garden carrot in warm water and took the drink to treat diabetes.*

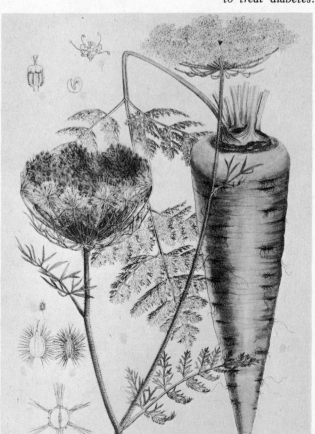

intake of carrots may lead to a condition known as carotinemia. The skin becomes yellowish, yielding a superficial resemblance to jaundice. This may explain why the Mohegan Indians associated carrots with liver disorders.

The carrot is put to many other interesting uses. The reddish juice was used as a natural food coloring; the syrup was made into a sweetening agent; French liqueurs are sometimes made with a tincture of carrot seed in alcohol; and carrot seed oil is used in perfumes. In times of shortage, roasted carrot roots have even substituted for coffee.

The wild relative of our garden carrots is very common in fields and waste places throughout North America. It grows between one and three feet high, and between May and September, it bears umbels of beautiful white flowers, the central one of each umbel often purple. It is sometimes called the bird's nest plant because before the lacy cluster of flowers appear, a hollow bird's-nest–shaped structure becomes apparent.

✑ DEVIL'S CLUB

It is not possible to know whether diabetes existed among the American Indians before the coming of the white man. That the disease does exist among many "full-blooded" American Indians today is verifiable. Perhaps following the early "doctrine of signatures," the Indians of British Columbia utilized a tea of the root bark of devil's club to offset the effects of diabetes. When tested clinically, it was discovered that an extract of this plant lowered the level of blood sugar in rabbits. How did these people learn to use devil's club for treating this metabolic upset?

This plant had long been used by the Thompson Indians of British Columbia to purify the blood and to serve as a tonic. This indicates that they may have been aware of the plant's effects on the liver. Other Coast Indians valued a decoction of the bark of this shrubby, prickly plant for its emetic effects. By vomiting, they purified themselves before a ceremony or important journey.

That devil's club had been used to treat diabetes in Indian medicine came to light around 1935 when an Indian was examined prior to an operation by a physician in British Columbia. Although the patient showed all the symptoms of this disease, he had survived for many years without medical care. When the doctor inquired, he learned that his Indian patient had kept himself in good health for years by drinking a root-bark tea of this interesting plant. This led to much discussion in medical circles and eventually to the experiments with rabbits.

This was the Coast Indians' second most important plant medicine; it also played an important role in their lore. They fashioned fishing hooks out of hemlock roots and attached a piece of devil's club bark to ensure a good catch of halibut. When attempting to persuade the gods, medicine men wore amulets of this wood. Partly because of its prickly stems, lodges for medicine men were constructed entirely of devil's club to keep these holy men sheltered from intruders.

DIARRHEA

This complaint is so common among all peoples that thousands of folk remedies have been evolved throughout the world to treat it. Diarrhea is a symptom of many diseases that are first manifested by a loose, and sometimes bloody, stool. The North American Indians utilized dozens of different plants to arrest this condition; some of the better-known species are listed below.

❦ BLACKBERRY (FIG.34)

A tea of blackberry roots was the most frequently used remedy for diarrhea among Indians of northern California. Five hundred Oneida Indians cured themselves of dysentery with this plant while the neighboring white settlers succumbed to the disease. The dried bark of the roots was official in the U.S. *Pharmacopoeia*, 1820 to 1916. It was also used for astringent purposes.

(FIG. 34) BLACKBERRY: *An entire village of Oneida Indians cured themselves of dysentery by drinking a root tea of this plant while the neighboring white settlers succumbed to the disease.*

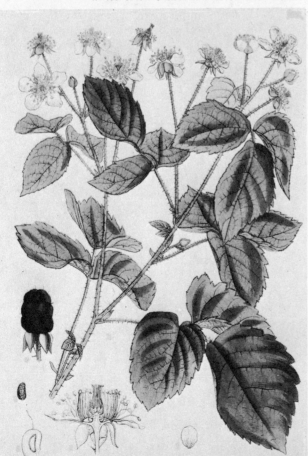

❦ CHOLLA CACTUS

Hopi chewed the raw cholla cactus root for diarrhea.

❦ RED CEDAR

Creeks and Choctaws drank oil from red cedar berries for dysentery.

❦ WILD BLACK CHERRY

The Mohegans allowed the ripe wild black cherry to ferment naturally in a jar for about one year and then drank the juice to cure dysentery. Wild cherry bark was listed in the U.S. *Pharmacopoeia* from 1820 to present. It was used as a sedative and in cough medicines.

❦ DOGWOOD

Menominees boiled the inner bark of the dogwood and passed the warm solution into the rectum with a rectal syringe composed of the bladder of a small mammal and the hollow bone of a bird. Dried bark of closely related species was listed in the U.S. *Pharmacopoeia* between 1820 and 1894 for astringent properties.

❦ SWEET FERN

The sweet fern was a very popular domestic remedy for diarrhea in the early 1900s. Leaves and flowering tops were boiled as a tea.

❦ GERANIUM

Chippewa and Ottawa tribes boiled the entire geranium plant and drank the tea for diarrhea. The dried rhizome was listed in the U.S. *Pharmacopoeia* from 1820 to 1916 as an astringent.

⋟ GREASEWOOD

The Pima Indians chewed and ingested the gum of the greasewood plant for dysentery. A gummy exudate was listed in the *U.S. Pharmacopoeia* from 1842 to 1942.

⋟ WHITE OAK

Iroquois and Penobscot boiled the bark of the white oak and drank the liquid for bleeding piles and diarrhea. It was once a very popular domestic remedy for diarrhea. The inner bark was listed in the *U.S. Pharmacopoeia* from 1820 to 1916 for astringent properties.

⋟ PERSIMMON

Cherokees drank a decoction of the boiled fruit of persimmon to treat bloody stools. The fruit was listed in the *U.S. Pharmacopoeia* from 1820 to 1882 as an astringent.

⋟ CUCKOW PINT

Iroquois boiled the bark of cuckow pint and drank the liquid for diarrhea.

⋟ BLACK RASPBERRY

The Pawnee, Omaha, and Dakota tribes boiled the root bark of black raspberry for dysentery. The fruit was listed in the *U.S. Pharmacopoeia* from 1882 to 1905 as a flavoring.

⋟ SENECA SNAKEROOT

Nishinam boiled the whole Seneca snakeroot plant and drank the liquid for diarrhea.

⋟ STAR GRASS

Catawbas drank a tea of star grass leaves for dysentery. The dried roots were listed in the *U.S. Pharmacopoeia* from 1820 to 1873 as a tonic.

DIGESTIVE DISORDERS

Disturbances of the digestive system were common among the American Indians due to their alternate periods of feasting and fasting. Long fasts were usually broken by great indulgence in large quantities of food, which placed great stress on the organs of digestion. Hundreds of remedies for treating "stomachache" appear in the literature. The following plants were selected for various reasons, some because they are well known, others because they were frequently employed, others because they were later accepted in "official" medicine for similar purposes, and still others to complete the geographical spectrum.

✑ BUTTERNUT (FIG. 35)

The Menominee Indians ate the syrup of the butternut, also called the white walnut, as a

(FIG. 35) BUTTERNUT: *The Menominee Indians ate the syrup of this "white walnut" as a standard remedy for digestive disorders.*

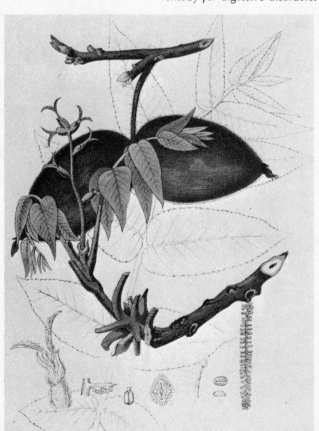

standard remedy for digestive disorders. The Potawatomis also drank a tea of the inner bark for stomach upsets, while the Meskwakis employed butternut bark in a tea as a mild laxative.

This plant, best known for its laxative properties, has been used in domestic American medicine for this purpose since before the Revolutionary War. It was especially valued as a laxative during the last century when some physicians thought it acted without colicky aftereffects. The inner root bark was official in the *U.S. Pharmacopoeia* from 1820 to 1905 when it was used for its laxative and tonic effects.

The leaves, bark, and unripe fruit yield a chocolate brown dye which was once an important coloring for woolens.

This tree, which belongs to the walnut family, grows between thirty and fifty feet in height. As illustrated, the sweet and oily nut is contained in a strong-smelling, sticky husk. These nuts are eaten fresh or stored for use in times of scarcity. The root bark was collected in autumn; around 1909, it was bringing the herb gatherer from one to four cents a pound.

✑ DANDELION (FIG. 36)

The common dandelion weed, so frequently eaten as a salad green and as a famine food, was also used in American Indian medicine soon after it was introduced to this country. No doubt the native Americans "borrowed" the recipes for this plant from the arriving European settlers.

A tea of the roots was drunk for heartburn by the Pillager Ojibwas, while the Mohegans and other tribes drank a tea of the leaves for their tonic properties. The dried rhizome and roots were official in the *U.S. Pharmacopoeia* from 1831 to 1926.

To verify the value of this common weed, we are told that many of the inhabitants of Minorca, one of the Balearic Islands, in the Mediterranean, subsisted on dandelion roots after their harvest had been entirely destroyed by locusts.

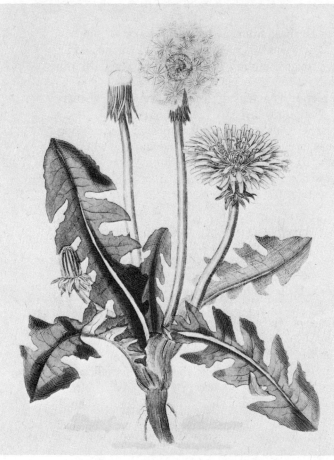

(FIG. 36) *DANDELION: This common weed, so frequently eaten as a salad green and as a famine food, was also used in American Indian medicine soon after it was introduced from Europe.*

❧ OREGON GRAPE

The state flower of Oregon, the Oregon grape, was used by the Kwakiutls of the northern Pacific Coast in the form of a bark tea to offset the digestive disorder characterized by an excess of bile. The Indians of California enjoyed a tea of the boiled roots as an apéritif.

The roots were soon adopted for domestic uses in America, and brisk trading at the beginning of this century almost exterminated the species around larger towns and cities.

The plant contains the alkaloid berberine; the roots were official in the *U.S. Pharmacopoeia* from 1905 to 1916 when they were used as a bitter tonic.

Oregon grape is indigenous to shady forests stretching from Colorado to the Pacific Ocean, being most abundant in Oregon and northern California. This low-growing shrub has three char-

acteristics that are easily observed: hollylike leaves; small, bright yellow flowers in April or May; and bluish berries that are pleasant to eat. When collecting the shrub for medicinal purposes, collectors were urged not to remove the bark from the rootstocks, probably in order to contain the moisture within thereby maintaining the roots' potency. The roots were gathered in the fall when they were richest in their chemical constituents.

❧ YELLOW ROOT

Interestingly, the same alkaloid that is present in Oregon grape root, berberine, is present in the yellow root. Yet an Indian tribe far removed from the Pacific Coast found similar uses for an unrelated species. How did the Catawba Indians of the North Carolina region come to discover tonic properties in the yellow root that were similar to the properties discovered in the root of the Oregon grape by the Coastal Indians?

This well-known Catawba and Cherokee "stomach" remedy was widely accepted among the white settlers; the rhizome and roots of yellow root were entered in the *U.S. Pharmacopoeia* from 1820 to 1882 when they were used for their tonic properties.

❧ SNOWBERRY

The following description of the fascinating snowberry bush was written by Thomas Jefferson in a letter to an aunt of Madame Lafayette, dated December 8, 1813.

> Lewis' journey across our continent to the Pacific has added a number of new plants to our former stock. Some of them curious, some ornamental, some useful, and some may by culture be made acceptable to our tables. I have growing, which I destine for you, a very handsome little shrub of the size of a currant bush. Its beauty consists in a great production of berries the size of currants, and literally as white as snow, which remain on the bush through the winter, after the leaves have fallen, and make it an object as singular as it is beautiful. We call it the snow-berry bush, no botanical name having yet been given it. (From Haskin, *Wild Flowers of the Pacific Coast*, p. 347)

The Thompson Indians of British Columbia boiled snowberry stems and drank the decoction for treating stomach problems. A weak solution of the stems was used as a wash for infants, while a stronger solution was applied to sores. In the late 1800s, the plant enjoyed some vogue in America as a remedy for vomiting in pregnancy.

The snowberry, which inhabits dry, open places, shows pink, bell-shaped flowers during June and July. The Pomo Indians of California described the slender, pithy stems as *sa-ka-hi*, or "wood for tobacco," because they fashioned this woody part into pipe stems.

✑§ STAR GRASS (FIG.37)

Star grass passed from the Catawba Indians to the herbalists and botanic-physicians who renamed the plant colic root in reference to its medicinal properties. The Indians had long used a tea of the leaves to treat all varieties of digestive disorders; it was adopted for its narcotic and tonic properties in American medicine, where the roots were used. The roots became official in the *U.S. Pharmacopoeia* in 1820, being continuously entered for their tonic properties until 1873.

Star grass grows in grassy woods throughout the eastern United States. The yellowish green leaves grow in a starlike cluster, and between May and August, a barren stalk appears that grows up to three feet in length. As illustrated, small white tubular flowers appear on the stem. The species name, *farinosa*, is from the Latin *farina*, which means "flour" and refers to the mealy texture of the blossoms.

The Thompson Indians sometimes boiled the bark of Rocky Mountain rhododendron and drank the tea for violent stomach upsets. They also used a root tea of wild ginger to relieve indigestion and colic.

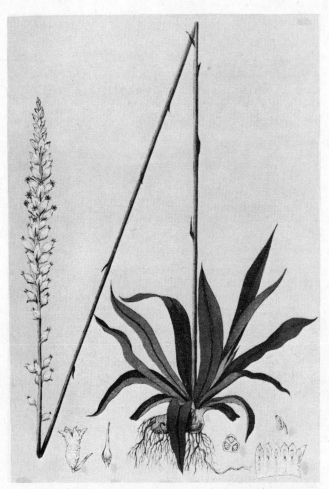

(FIG. 37) STAR GRASS: *Star grass passed from the Catawba Indians to the herbalists who renamed the plant colicroot in reference to its medicinal properties.*

EARACHE

Since the effects of all the following plants are treated elsewhere in this book and the following treatments were probably of scant therapeutic value, Indian treatments for earache will merely be enumerated.

✒ MESCAL BEAN

The Kickapoo Indians of Wisconsin used to crush mescal beans, boil them in water, strain off the particles, and then pour the liquid into aching ears.

✒ WILD GINGER

The Meskwakis steeped the pounded wild ginger root and poured the liquid into the ear. The dried rhizome and roots of this species were in the *U.S. Pharmacopoeia* from 1820 to 1873, and it has been reported by Vogel and others that two antibiotic substances have been found in this drug.

✒ WILD LICORICE

Wild licorice leaves were steeped in water and the resulting liquid then used for earache by the Blackfoot Indians.

✒ WHITE MILKWORT

White milkwort root was scraped, then boiled in water, and the resulting liquid poured into aching ears by the Sioux.

✒ TOBACCO (FIG. 38)

The Rappahannock, Mohegan, and Malecite Indians blew tobacco smoke into the ear as a cure. The leaves were official in the *U.S. Pharmacopoeia* from 1820 to 1905 when they were used

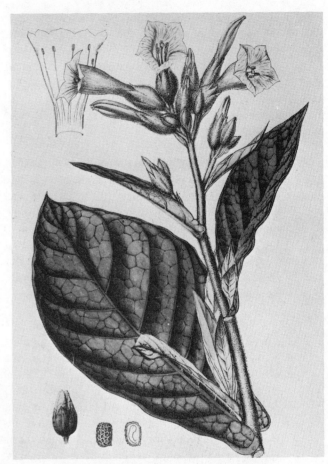

(FIG. 38) TOBACCO: *Several tribes blew tobacco smoke into the ear as a cure for earache.*

for narcotic and sedative purposes. Times and plant uses certainly change!

✒ YARROW

The Winnebagos steeped the whole yarrow plant and poured the resulting liquid into the ear. The dried leaves and tops of yarrow, listed in the *U.S. Pharmacopoeia* from 1863 to 1882, were used for promoting menstruation and for their stimulant properties.

EPILEPSY

As another investigator has shown, epilepsy was not common among the aboriginal Indians. Several "cures" are reported, but these were usually performed for white patients by an Indian practitioner. With the exception of the cow parsnip, the other species used for treatment are discussed elsewhere in this book and will only be listed here.

◆§ COW PARSNIP

Cow parsnip roots have a strong and disagreeable odor and cause redness and inflammation when brought in contact with the skin. Resembling the roots of parsley, they were used by the Ojibwas, Menominees, and Meskwakis as an external application on sores and wounds, for cramps and headache, and in ritual, respectively.

Eclectic physicians used this species for epilepsy; however, only stimulant and carminative properties are listed in the *Dispensatory of the United States.* The eclectics chose the form of therapy which they thought would be most beneficial for any one patient and maintained that treatment program throughout the course of his illness. This group of physicians, which commonly employed plant remedies, borrowed heavily from American Indian remedies.

Although not much else is known regarding the use of cow parsnip in treating epilepsy, it is a useful food. When the young leaf stalks and stems are boiled in two changes of water, they make a tasty celerylike vegetable. Some Indians peeled the stalks and ate them raw, while the large root, considered poisonous by some authors, was cooked and eaten as a potato.

This coarse, umbelliferous plant grows in moist soils, such as in the marshy thickets extending from northern North America to North Carolina. It grows as high as six to eight feet and bears large umbels of white flowers. The thick stem divides into three main divisions, each bearing coarse, large leaves which are wooly on the lower surface.

The Creek Indians prepared a large bath of the roots of boneset in boiling water and immersed the epileptic in the rising steam. Although passionflower is treated under "Sedatives," it should be noted here that this species was included in a list of native American botanical medicines compiled in 1783 by a visiting European physician. This visitor merely mentioned that the plant was used in epilepsy without commenting on the effects, etc. Indians used passionflower for swellings, sore eyes, and to induce vomiting. It has been shown that an extract of the plant depresses the motor nerves of the spinal cord.

EYE PROBLEMS

MESQUITE

The thin membrane which protects the eye-ball was frequently irritated in the eyes of those Indians who lived in dwellings that were usually filled with smoke. Thus, we find reports which indicate that many teepee dwellers suffered from irritated conjunctiva.

Mesquite has long been a favorite eye lotion among the Indians of the Southwest. These tribes probably learned about the plant from Indians of South America because Vogel shows that the Aztecs called this species *mizquitl* and prepared an eye medicine from the leaves. The Mescalero Apaches, Pimas, and Maricopas all used various parts of this herb to treat sore and painful eye membranes. The Apaches added water to the powdered leaves and then squeezed the liquid through a cloth on the eyes. Another tribe applied the sap directly on the inflammed lids.

Mesquite is a large shrub or low tree with arched branches and forked leaves. The tiny flowers are arranged in small spikes, and the characteristic pods are from two to six inches long. This species is common throughout the Southwest where the fruit contained in the compressed pod is a useful survival food. This sweet pulpy interior, which is 30 percent grape sugar, was eaten by the Indians of that region fresh or cooked in water.

INDIAN PIPE (FIG.39)

The Indian pipe is a plant whose corpselike, bluish waxy appearance attracted the imagination of an early Indian herb doctor and led him to try mixing its juices with water as a medicine for "sore eyes." This remedy obviously "caught on" because it was soon being used throughout its geographical range to cure eye irritations.

This strange, ghostlike plant was also known as corpse plant because of its resemblance to the dead. It is cool and clammy to the touch and

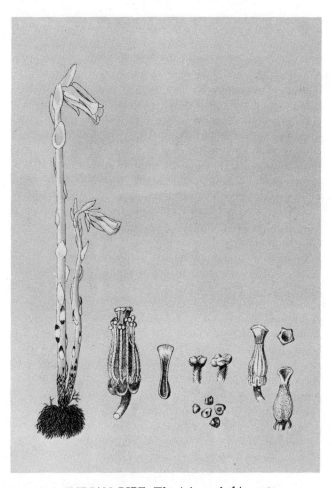

(FIG. 39) INDIAN PIPE: *The juices of this corpse-like, bluish, waxy plant were widely used to cure eye irritations.*

readily decays and turns black when touched. This ghoul of the plant world contains no chlorophyll and derives its nourishment from decaying vegetable matter in the earth. It bears a solitary flower between June and October and thrives in deep, rich, shady woods from Florida to Mississippi but also extends northward to Alaska in scattered areas.

When used for eye problems, the plant was bruised and the clear fluid of the stems applied.

A Dr. Kunze describes his experiences with Indian pipe in the *Botanical Gazette* for 1878,

Fourteen years ago . . . I went woodcock shooting with two friends, near Hackensack, N.J., and while taking some luncheon in a beech grove along the course of Saddle River, I found a large patch of . . . *Monotropa uniflora* in full bloom . . . a beautiful sight of snow-white stems and nodding flowers . . . I proceeded to fill my game-bag, and to the question, what it was used for, answered: "Good for sore eyes," little thinking that the party addressed was suffering from a chronic inflammation of the eye-lids, the edges of which had a very fiery-red appearance . . . he made very good use of it . . . his inflamed lids were entirely cured in four weeks time . . . by applying the fresh juice of the stems. . . .

The Blackfoot Indians treated sore eyes with several different preparations. One consisted of the leaves and flowers of yarrow steeped in fresh water; other eye washes were made from the leaves of the snowberry or from the flowers of the horsemint. Another Blackfoot eye wash consisted of a decoction of the roots of the prairie smoke plant.

There were many other eye preparations used by various tribes; only a few of these are listed below. The Gosiute Indians steeped the leaves of western ragweed; the Paiute and Shoshoni made a poultice of the fresh, crushed leaves of blue flax; the Pima Indians steeped pluchia leaves; and the Indians of the Missouri River region steeped the leaves of the Indian currant.

FEVERS

⇝ BAYBERRY (FIG. 40)

The bayberry is best known for the wax that is obtained from its berries and used for making candles. Although its bark enjoyed some popularity in domestic American medicine for its astringent and tonic properties, the root bark was official in the *National Formulary* for only twenty years, from 1916 to 1936.

The wax which forms around the berries was also used medicinally. It was boiled "to an extract [as] a certain cure for the most violent cases of dysentery." Some physicians of the eighteenth century even considered this wax a narcotic!

For candle making, bayberry fruits are boiled in water until the wax floats; it is then skimmed off with a spoon, strained of impurities, and boiled a second time. Millspaugh stated:

Candles made from this wax, though quite brittle, are less greasy in warm weather, of fine appearance, slightly aromatic, and smokeless after snuffing, rendering them much more pleasant to use than those made of either wax or tallow. Soap from this wax makes an aromatic and very softening shaving lather and a fine body for surgeons' soap plasters.

Indian use of this plant was quite limited. Only one tribe, the Louisiana Choctaws, employed it as a fever remedy. They boiled the leaves and stems and drank the resulting tea.

Bayberry is found in swampy regions throughout the southeastern states. It varies in size in its different geographies. In its southernmost limits, it is a small evergreen tree attaining a maximum height of forty feet, but in the northern perimeter of its growing range, it becomes a small shrub about three feet high. It has a smooth gray bark, leaves that are fragrant when crushed, and yellowish flowers. The bluish white berries, which are the source of the greenish white wax, remain on the tree for years.

⇝ DOGWOOD (FIG. 41)

Dogwood is an old Indian remedy for fever. The Delaware Indians, who called the tree *Hatta-wa-no-min-schi*, boiled the inner bark in water, employing the tea to reduce fevers. The bark of flowering dogwood was similarly employed by the Alabamas and the Houmas of Louisiana.

During the last century, cinchona bark, which is an important source of quinine, was the most efficacious remedy for malarial fevers. Imported from Peru, it remained largely unobtainable to residents of the southern states during the American Civil War. At that time, flowering dogwood was substituted for Peruvian barks as a fever remedy.

Various species of dogwood have appeared in several editions of the *U.S. Pharmacopoeia*; however, the glucoside cornin, which is contained within the bark, is presently recognized only for its astringent properties.

This small forest tree grows between ten and thirty feet high and has grayish bark on the trunk and reddish bark on the branches. The snowy

(FIG. 40) BAYBERRY: *The Louisiana Choctaws boiled the stems and leaves of this famous wax plant and drank the resulting tea as a fever remedy.*

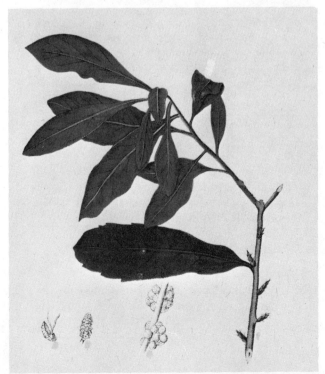

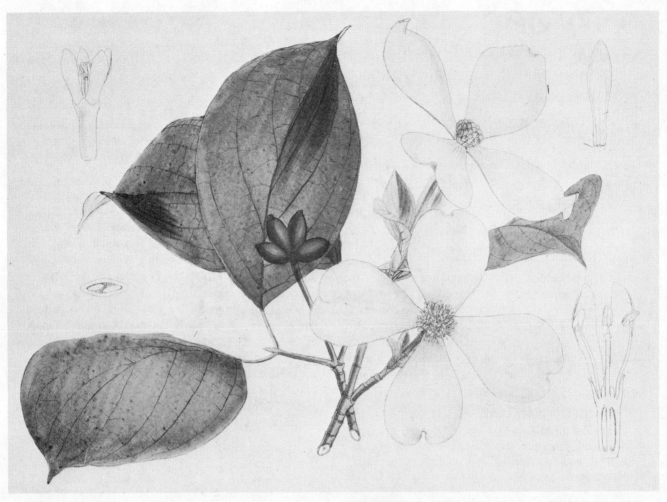

(FIG. 41) DOGWOOD: *The Alabamas and the Houmas of Louisiana boiled the inner bark of this small forest tree in water and drank the resulting tea to reduce fevers.*

white flowers, which appear in the spring, are followed by a few red berrylike fruits that contain a two-seeded nutlet.

~§ TREE OF HEAVEN

The large tree of heaven was not employed by the Indians, but it did cause a great deal of controversy in this country soon after its introduction from China. It is included in this work for the very interesting application it was assigned by the masses. This may serve as an example of the state of our "scientific medicine" only one hundred and fifty years ago. Millspaugh describes it in his work *American Medicinal Plants*:

The *Ailanthus* tree was introduced into England in the year 1751, and thrived well; about the year 1800 it was brought to this country, and soon grew in public favor as an ornamental tree for lawns, walks and streets; later on it became in greater demand on account of its supposed property of absorbing from the atmosphere malarial poisons; under this new idea the tree became a great favorite in cities and large towns, especially as its growth was rapid and its beautiful foliage pleasing. The occurrence, however, of several severe epidemics, especially in the larger cities, set people thinking—might not this tree, which so fully absorbs poison, also throw off toxic effluvia? May it not store up the noxious gases and again set them forth in the flowering season? . . . A war upon the trees followed, both wordy and actual, which almost banished them from the country.

~§ WHITE OR SILVER POPLAR

Salicin, the febrifuge and analgesic glucoside discussed at greater length in the section on the willow, is obtained from the bark of this poplar species.

Several Indian tribes reportedly treated themselves with parts of this tree, and the bark was entered in the *U.S. Pharmacopoeia* from 1895 to 1936 when the salicin it contains was used to reduce fever and to relieve the pain of menstrual cramps.

ᴥ§ JOE-PYE WEED

Joe Pye was an Indian practitioner from New England who gained fame by curing typhus with the joe-pye weed. Closely related to boneset (see "Colds"), it was used in a number of ways by several Indian tribes.

The Iroquois drank a tea of the leaves to promote the flow of urine (diuretic), the main use to which the joe-pye weed was put in domestic American medicine.

ᴥ§ WILLOW (FIG. 42)

Most of the willows have been used for their pain-relieving and fever-lowering properties since the time of Dioscorides, the ancient Greek physician (circa A.D. 60) who investigated and described six hundred species of plants and their medicinal properties. In 1763, the bark was recommended specifically for fevers and enjoyed tremendous popularity in America. The fresh bark contains salicin, which probably decomposes into salicylic acid in the human system. Aspirin, a well-known drug taken for its analgesic and febrifuge effects, is chemically related to salicylic acid. The structural formulas for each are shown below.

ASPIRIN (Acetylsalicylic acid)   SALICYLIC ACID (from willow bark)

Whether the Indians learned to utilize the indigenous black willow independent of the arriving European who brought with him knowledge of the medicinal properties of the white willow is not clear.

Willows were employed throughout their range

of growth in the United States. Thus, the Pomo tribe boiled the inner root bark of the willow tree found in California (western willow). These Indians drank strong doses of the resulting tea to promote sweating in cases of chills and fever. In

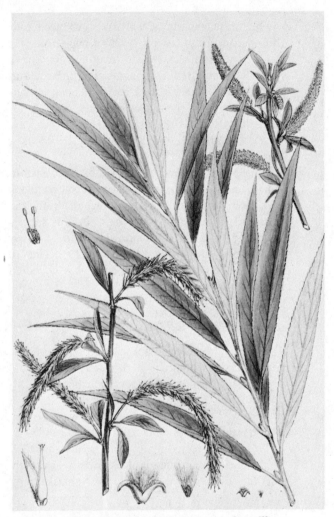

(FIG. 42) WHITE WILLOW: *Most of the willows have been used for their fever-lowering properties since the time of Dioscorides, the ancient Greek physician. Many Indian tribes of North America boiled the inner bark and drank the tea in strong doses to relieve pain and to reduce fevers.*

the south, the Natchez prepared their fever remedies from the bark of the red willow, while the Alabama and Creek Indians plunged into willow root steam baths for the same purpose. The use of willow is also reported among the Pima of Arizona, the Houma of Mississippi, the Mohegans of Connecticut, the Penobscots of Maine, the

Montagnais of southeastern Canada, and several other American tribes.

The glucoside salicin, as obtained from various species of willow, was official in the U.S. *Pharmacopoeia* from 1882 through 1926. It has since been superseded by aspirin and other synthetic preparations.

The white willow, which was introduced into this country from Europe, occurs along streams in the northeastern states. It sometimes attains a height of ninety feet, has rough grayish bark, and as illustrated, lance-shaped leaves. The long catkins appear with the leaves in the spring. As an emergency food, the bast, or woody cells, are sometimes ground into a flour and baked as a "bread."

The pussy willow, a native of the eastern United States, has rough, dark brown or black bark and yellowish, brittle branches. Both the bark and catkins (pussy willows) of this species have been used in medicine. The bark is easily removed in the spring when the sap begins to flow; this was the season when it was collected for the drug market.

✑§ FEVERWORT (FIG.43)

The Cherokees drank a decoction of the coarse, leafy, perennial herb feverwort to cure fevers. The rhizome and roots, which contain an alkaloid, were employed in domestic practice as cathartics. Following this usage, it was used in treating inflammatory fevers by the eclectics.

This indigenous herb prefers the shade of forests and a limestone soil. It is dispersed throughout the eastern states, west to Nebraska, and blossoms in June.

There were some other fever-relieving plants utilized by various tribes. The Cheyennes drank a febrifuge tea prepared from the finely ground leaves and stems of silver-leaf psoralea steeped in

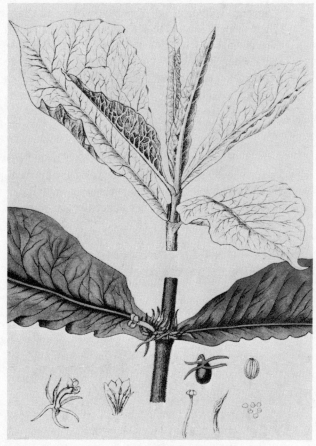

(FIG. 43) *FEVERWORT: The Cherokees drank a strong tea made of this coarse leafy herb to cure fevers.*

boiling water. The Cherokees and Natchez preferred the Virginia snakeroot to any other plant used for treating high fevers. The first-named tribe boiled the root while the other steeped the whole plant.

To treat fevers in the northwestern United States, the Blackfoot Indians drank a tea of the steeped bee plant or used an infusion of the white bark of the western clematis. These people sometimes also boiled the root bark of creeping mahonia.

FROSTBITE

There are few reported incidents of frostbite among the American Indians. This is true because those who ventured far from their fellows and were frozen probably died. Of course, this may not have been important enough among the Indians to have been spoken about. What serves as a major personal catastrophe in our culture may well have been completely accepted and little discussed by the American Indian.

In addition to protectively insulating themselves with animal fats and oils, the Indians utilized a few plant remedies for treating frostbite. A decoction of the boiled leaves of white beech was sometimes poured over the affected part, as was a leaf decoction of smooth upland sumac. Plasters of the resin of various pines were similarly used on the frozen member.

The Chippewas amputated gangrenous limbs that originated from severe frostbite and applied a poultice of the pounded bark of the wild black cherry to the amputee's limb stump.

HAIR

Individuals of the Thompson tribe of British Columbia reported that their people had excellent hair when they had used hair washes made from wild plants. They believed that the use of commercial soaps caused their hair to dry out and turn gray prematurely. Of course, it is possible that the entire cultural change, including the incorporation of the new products manufactured great distances from their native environment, caused this "premature graying." Some of the hair washes used by the Thompsons and other tribes are listed below.

The Hopi Indians steeped the leaves of Apache plume and applied the liquid as a rinse to promote hair growth. The Blackfoot tribe soaked the leaves of winter fat in warm water for a hair wash or alternately used the pounded roots of soaproot as a wash.

The scouring rush (FIG.44) was used in many ways by Indians of the western states. The stalks were boiled by the Washington Indians, and the resulting decoction employed as a hair wash to eliminate fleas, lice, and mites. To cure diarrhea, the heads of the reproductive shoots were eaten by the Makah tribe. This fern was also used ceremonially, while the tough stalk was employed as an abrasive for scouring and sharpening arrows and mussel shells.

Although the ferns which belong to the horsetail family were little used in American medicine, the field horsetail contains equisetic acid which is thought to be identical with aconitic acid. This substance is a potent heart and nerve sedative that is a dangerous poison when taken in high doses. Other members of the genus contain equisetine, an alkaloid that has been responsible for poisoning in livestock.

The Indians of California prepared a hair wash from the steeped fronds of the wood fern, a member of the polypodium family of ferns. This tribe sometimes treated cuts with the pulverized roots of the same species.

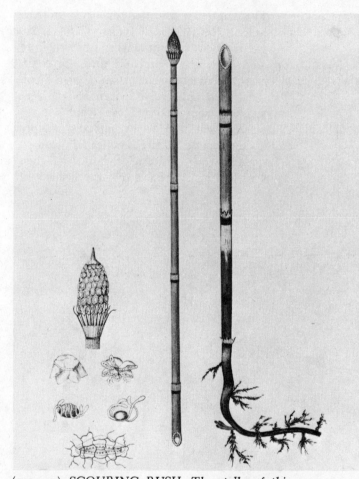

(FIG. 44) SCOURING RUSH: The stalks of this fern were boiled and the liquid employed as a hair wash to eliminate fleas, lice, and mites by the Washington Indians.

In the Northwest, the Thompson tribe boiled the entire blue Jacob's-ladder plant and used the liquid decoction as a hair rinse. They also made washes of tobacco and of blue flax.

Another hair wash was prepared by boiling the columbine plant. The scarlet flowers bear large stores of honey which are often eaten by hungry hikers. The roots were boiled and eaten as a famine food by the Indians of the western states.

HEADACHE

ᴁ SKUNK CABBAGE (FIG.45)

The foul-smelling skunk cabbage weed was formerly employed in American medicine as an emetic, diuretic, and antispasmodic drug. The roots and rhizome were used in treating various respiratory and nervous disorders; they were official in the U.S. *Pharmacopoeia* from 1880 to 1882.

Indian usage of this species was quite limited. Of the six or so tribes that used the skunk cabbage, only the Micmacs specifically treated headache with it. They bound a bunch of the leaves together, crushed them, and inhaled the sharp odor. This plant hardly meets the requirements to be listed as a "representative" Indian headache remedy, but it is included because it is interesting to note that a plant which is presently avoided because of its rank odor was once inhaled to *cure* headache.

Perhaps the Micmacs used the skunk cabbage *because* it has such a trying odor. This would fit the "doctrine of signatures," where "like cures like." Perhaps the Micmacs thought that if smelling a plant could induce a headache in a healthy person, smelling the same plant could cure a sick person.

This member of the arum family inhabits swamps and other wet places throughout the eastern United States and west to Iowa. The hood-shaped, purplish flowers appear before the leaves, in February or March. The large leaves are borne on thick stems. When it was used in medicine, the rootstock was collected in the early spring or late fall. It was never stored for a long time because the properties appear to diminish with age.

ᴁ PENNYROYAL (FIG.46)

The Onondagas, a divisional tribe of the mighty Iroquois, steeped pennyroyal leaves and

(FIG. 45) SKUNK CABBAGE: *The Micmacs bound the leaves of this plant together, crushed them, and inhaled the sharp odor to cure headaches.*

(FIG. 46) PENNYROYAL: *The Onondagas, a divisional tribe of the Iroquois, steeped pennyroyal leaves and drank the tea to cure headaches.*

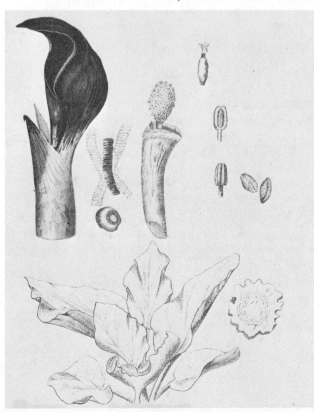

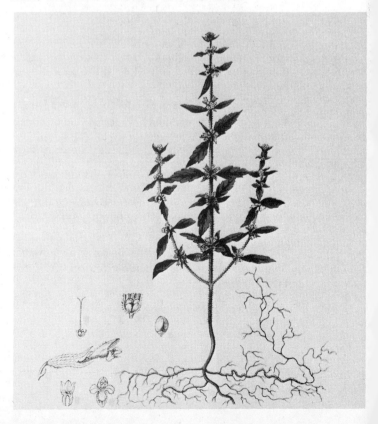

drank the resulting tea to cure headaches. In the western states, the Mescalero Apaches used a related species (*H. reverchoni*) for headache by crushing the twigs and inhaling the mintlike odor.

Pennyroyal was extensively used in domestic American medicine to induce sweating in the early stages of colds, to promote menstruation, with brewer's yeast to induce abortion, and with raw linseed oil to dress burns. The dried leaves were official in the *U.S. Pharmacopoeia* from 1831 to 1916.

This aromatic herb is found in dry soil in southeastern Canada and the eastern United States, west to the Dakotas. The plant seldom grows above one foot in height. It has small, opposite leaves on short stems and a few pale blue flowers, which appear from July to September. When collected for the drug market, pennyroyal leaves and flowering tops were gathered while in flower and the volatile oil of pennyroyal distilled from them.

❧ INDIAN TURNIP (FIG.47)

The wild Indian turnip was used by several tribes, but only the Pawnee Indians powdered the root and applied it to the head and temples to cure headache. Indian headache remedies usually took one of three forms: a tea of a particular plant part, an inhalant formed by crushing a succulent plant, or, as in the case of the Indian turnip, a dusting powder made by drying and pulverizing the root.

The *Dispensatory of the United States* says that freshly dug Indian turnip roots are dangerous and intensely acrid, while roots which have been thoroughly dried are inactive. For these reasons the fresh, partially dried roots were used in medicine to stimulate secretions in asthma, rheumatism, and whooping cough. The corm was official in the *U.S. Pharmacopoeia* from 1820 to 1893.

Although we are cautioned against eating the Indian turnip because of the calcium oxalate it contains, the Indians wisely pounded the roots to a pulp with water and allowed the mass to dry for several weeks before using it as a source of flour. This process is said to destroy the acrid taste.

Indian turnip is found in moist woods in the eastern states from Florida north to Canada and west to Minnesota. The plant grows between one and three feet in height, and the green and brownish purple hooded flowers appear in April. As illustrated, the leaves are borne on long, erect

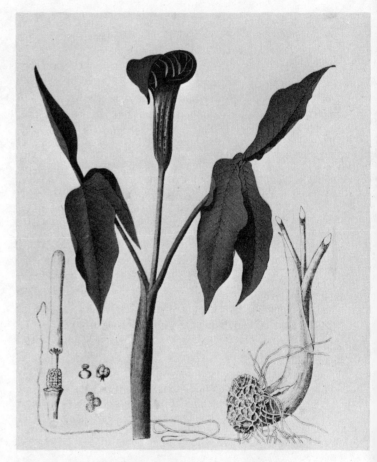

(FIG. 47) INDIAN TURNIP: *The powdered root of this plant was applied to the head and temples by the Pawnees to cure headaches.*

stalks and consist of three leaflets. The hooded "flower," known as a spathe, shelters the club-shaped spadix. In the fall, bright scarlet berries are formed, but these too are acrid.

Many, many other plants were employed to cure this too-common malady, and a few of them are listed below. The Montagnais tribe crushed buttercup leaves and inhaled the odor; the Meskwakis prepared a tea of anemone roots for headache and dizziness; the Ojibwas drank a tea of the leaves of white cedar; the Choctaws pounded elder leaves and mixed them with salt before applying the mass to the head; the Chickasaws soaked red cedar limbs in warm water with elder and applied the wet limbs on the head. In the Southwest, the Zuñi steeped a variety of lamb's-quarters in hot water and inhaled the steam as a headache remedy.

Finally, we come to an old Zuñi medicine that was originally used to hasten childbirth and later became an accepted substitute for ergot, which has been prescribed for headache in American medicine. The Zuñis dissolved a very small quantity of the fungus *Ustilago zeae* that grows upon the stems and flowers of Indian corn, and drank the infusion to induce labor. This fungus contains an alkaloid, ustilagine, which has been used in medicine like ergot—to promote uterine contractions, and in migraine, to constrict the blood vessels of the scalp or brain thereby reducing the flow of blood and relieving the throbbing effect that accompanies each heartbeat. This fungus was official in the *U.S. Pharmacopoeia* from 1882 to 1894, which is a great credit to the Zuñi practitioners who discovered its usefulness by their own inspired methods.

HEART AND CIRCULATORY PROBLEMS

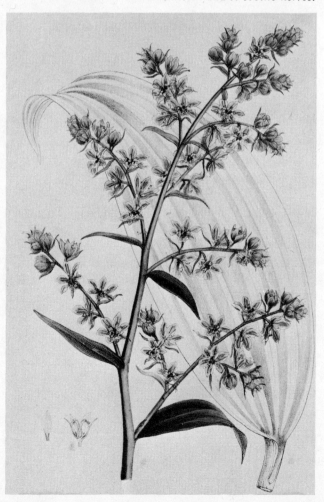

GREEN HELLEBORE (FIG.48)

The Cherokee Indians used the green hellebore to relieve body pains, while the Thompson tribe of British Columbia boiled the roots of a related species (V. *californicum*) and drank a small quantity of the decoction for syphilis and disorders of the blood.

(FIG. 48) GREEN HELLEBORE: *Several tribes used this plant for various complaints; however, it was the early settlers who first used it to slow the heart's action and to soothe nerves.*

John Josselyn, an early explorer of America, observed that in 1638, the root was used by the young Indian braves in an ordeal to choose the chiefs; "he whose stomach withstood its action the longest was decided to be the strongest of the party, and entitled to command the rest."

Green hellebore was boiled by the early settlers, and the decoction used as a wash to destroy lice, fleas, etc.

The dried rhizome and roots were later employed in medicine to slow the heart's action and to soothe nerves. The plant contains the alkaloids jervine, pseudo-jervine, and veratridine, and several other minor constituents. The *Dispensatory of the United States* for 1942 finds this plant "a very valuable agent for the reduction of blood pressure in various conditions of hypertension." This is quite a statement coming from a publication that is generally skeptical about plant medicines.

Green hellebore was official in the *U.S. Pharmacopoeia* from 1820 to 1942, and in the *National Formulary* from 1942 to 1960. It was used to lower blood pressure, to depress the heart's action, and to soothe nerves, but has since been superseded by synthetic agents.

Green hellebore is found growing in moist meadows throughout the eastern and central United States. Its range extends through Canada to Alaska. The bright green leaves appear early in spring and are followed by a stout, erect stem which grows as high as six feet. The leaves are very large and broadly oval and have distinct parallel veins. The greenish yellow flowers, which are borne in open clusters, appear from May to July. When used for medicine, the rootstock was dug in autumn after the leaves were dead. This plant is sometimes confused with the edible skunk cabbage, but must not be eaten because the alkaloids are quite poisonous.

◆§ AMERICAN HEMP AND DOGBANE
(FIG.49)

The native American hemp and dogbane species were utilized first in American Indian medicine and then later recognized and accepted by the American medical profession. Interestingly, these species have been found to contain a drug that is closely related to digitalis, the widely used cardiotonic drug.

Dogbane was long used by the Prairie Potawatomis as a heart medicine. The fruit was boiled when it was still green, and the resulting decoction drunk. It was also used for kidney problems and for dropsy, a condition characterized by an accumulation of fluid in the tissues. This fluid retention is usually due to heart or kidney failure. Since it has been shown that these plants act by regulating and strengthening the heart's action, it is easy to speculate that the Indian practitioner had a good understanding of the circulatory system, and selected those plants of his environment which would restore balance to a faltering unit.

This may not be the case. Eric Stone, the physician-author who researched *Medicine among the American Indians*, states in his book that they did not know very much about the heart and circulatory system. Although many tribes were able to distinguish between veins and arteries and knew that the flow of arterial blood was caused by the heart, it is nowhere suggested that they understood the relationship between a failing heart and the collection of water in the tissues. But since our knowledge of the aboriginal Indians is certainly less complete than was their knowledge of the circulatory system, we can't be sure about what they knew.

In any case, both the dogbane and American hemp were official in the *U.S. Pharmacopoeia*. The *Dispensatory of the United States* states that both species are "used as a substitute for digitalis in the treatment of chronic heart disease" and that "in moderate dose causes a slowing of the pulse and increase in the amplitude of the cardiac contractions. . . ." The one drawback to clinical use, we learn, is that the drug irritates the intestines and may cause very unsatisfactory side effects.

Like most plants of the family, American hemp contains a milky juice. This herb is commonly found in thickets, along fences, and over old fields. It attains a height of two to four feet and bears small greenish white flowers in dense heads from June to August. These are followed by the characteristic slender pods which are about four inches in length and pointed at the tips. When used in medicine, the root of American hemp was collected in the fall. The bark was also made into twine and fishing nets by the Indians and has been sewed for sails. The milky latex of this species was even utilized as a source of chewing gum by the Kiowas.

Indian hemp, or marijuana, (FIG.50) is not botanically related to the American hemp, nor is it pharmacologically similar. However, marijuana was at one time an official drug in the U.S. *Pharmacopoeia* and was regularly used wherever a sedative, analgesic, or narcotic drug was required. Bear in mind that the medical definition for *narcotic* is an "agent that produces stupor or sleep."

Owing to the present interest in this plant, an illustration drawn by Dr. Millspaugh from specimens "growing at Union, N.Y., [on] July

(FIG. 49) DOGBANE: *The green fruit was boiled by the prairie Potawatomis who drank the resulting liquid as a heart medicine.*

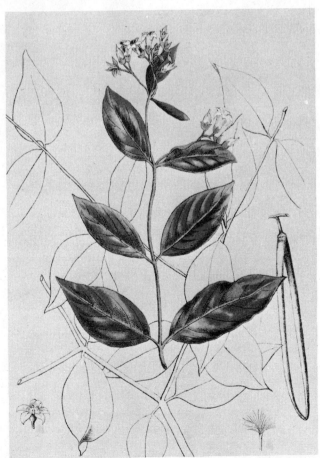

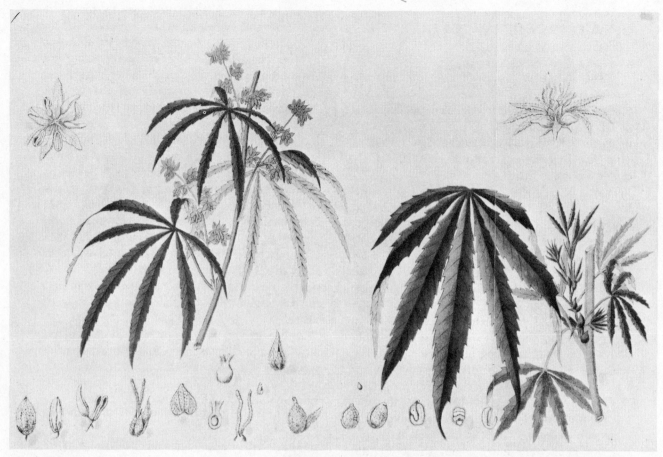

(FIG. 50) MARIJUANA: *This infamous weed was not used by the American Indians but it was at one time an official drug in the* United States Pharmacopoeia *and was regularly used wherever a sedative, analgesic, or narcotic was required.*

26, 1886" is included. It may also be of interest to read how marijuana was employed when it was used in general practice:

the drug is used wherever an anodyne, hypnotic, or antispasmodic is judged necessary; the various diseases where it proves effectual are hardly mentionable, as the benefit is almost always homoeopathic, therefore, each disease should be individualized. Surgical tetanus, gonorrhoea, leucorrhoea, inflammation of the mucous membranes of the bladder and urethra, dysuria, delirium, and melancholia may be, however, mentioned as the diseases in which our Old School brothers usually get the most decided effects from this drug.

Before leaving this species and returning to heart medicines used by the American Indians, I would like to complete Dr. Millspaugh's observations on marijuana by quoting from his section on "physiological action" of the plant in tincture and infusion. The following effects were compiled by five physicians who administered the drug to an unstated number of subjects.

Depression and absent-mindedness; confusion, vertigo, and congestion, followed by cephalalgia; earache; toothache; dryness of the mouth, throat and lips; loss of appetite; nausea, and vomiting after coffee; slight inflammation of the meatus urinarius, and diminished urine; sexual excitement without desire; oppression of the chest, and palpitation of the heart; weakness of the limbs; itching of the skin; and dreaminess during sleep.

To give this diversion an international flavor, I include a discussion of the medical properties and uses of marijuana as stated in Bentley's series on *Medicinal Plants* which was published in London in 1880. The plant was, at that time, official in the *Pharmacopoeias* of Britain and India.

Indian Hemp produces a peculiar kind of intoxication, attended with exhilaration of the spirits and hallucinations, said to be generally of a pleasing kind. These are followed by narcotic effects, sleep and stupor. In its anodyne and soporific action it resembles opium, but its aftereffects are considered less unpleasant; it does not produce constipation nor loss of appetite. Indian hemp possesses antispasmodic and anodyne powers, for which it has been chiefly employed in medicine. It has been administered in the different forms of neuralgia, in spasmodic coughs, as pertussis and asthma, also in tetanus, hydrophobia, and other anomalous spasmodic and painful diseases. Sometimes, but very seldom, it has been used to procure sleep.

WAHOO (FIG.51)

The native wahoo shrub was used in Indian medicine for a variety of purposes (uterine prob-

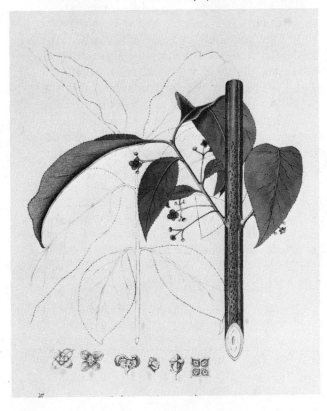

(FIG. 51) WAHOO: *This native shrub was borrowed from the Indians and soon became a popular diuretic drug. It exerts a digitalislike effect on the heart and at one time was a popular heart medicine.*

lems, as a physic, as an eye wash, etc.); however, soon after its introduction to the early settlers, the bark became a popular diuretic drug. It was not until a report was published in 1912 which showed that this species effects a digitalislike action on the heart that wahoo became a popular heart medicine in domestic practice.

Wahoo is found in moist, open woods, and along rivers from the eastern United States west to Montana. It grows between six and twenty-five feet in height and has gray bark and opposite leaves. Its purple flowers appear in June, and the pale purple fruits are produced in October. After this time, the fruits burst open and give a fiery appearance which is especially apparent if this occurs after the leaves have fallen and the wahoo is encountered against a snow background. It is due to this appearance in winter that the plant has also been called the burning bush.

When used in medicine, wahoo bark, which has a sweetish taste, was gathered in the fall. It should be noted that although the attractive fruits have sometimes been eaten, they are considered poisonous by some writers and should definitely be avoided.

The following species were used as cardiac stimulants: Holly was steeped and the infusion drunk by North Carolina Indians; horsemint was used by the Winnebago and Dakota tribes; and bush morning-glory was taken by the Pawnee Indians.

To relieve heart palpitations, the Canadian Indians drank an infusion of wild ginger, while the Catawbas used the same plant to relieve heart pains. The Flambeau Ojibwas utilized a tea made by steeping a species of violet to treat "heart problems," as did the Potawatomis. The Indians of Nevada and Utah even used a root decoction of alum to treat heart disorders.

If the reader is not confused by this list of very, very diverse plants which were considered heart medicines by equally diverse tribes of Indians, read through the list of concoctions that were devised to treat hemorrhoids (piles).

HEMORRHOIDS

⊷ WHITE OAK

Of the more than fifty species of oak found in the United States, the white oak has been the most important medicinal species, both to the Indians and to the whites. Oak bark contains from six to eleven percent tannin, the agent that gives it its property of drying up body tissues.

The Indians recognized the astringent properties of oak bark and used it mainly for treating diarrhea, dysentery, cuts, and piles.

The Menominee tribe treated piles by squirting an infusion of the scraped inner bark of oak into the rectum with a syringe made from an animal bladder and the hollow bone of a bird. This type of syringe was commonly made by many tribes. It appears in the literature as also having been used by the Penobscots and Iroquois to squirt an oak bark infusion into the rectum to cure bloody piles.

The inner bark of white oak, used for astringent, tonic, and antiseptic purposes in American medicine, was official in the *U.S. Pharmacopoeia* from 1820 to 1916.

In addition to being a useful medicinal agent, this tree furnishes a tough, strong wood that has been used in construction and in the manufacture of furniture, railroad ties, fences, baskets, and agricultural tools.

The white oak is found throughout the eastern and central United States, being most abundant in the middle of the country. This stately tree sometimes grows as high as one hundred and fifty feet, but is more commonly about sixty to eighty feet in height with a trunk diameter of three to four feet. The bark is scaly and gray, and the leaves and acorns typical. In the fall the leaves turn a beautiful red. When used for its tannin, the inner bark of white oak was collected in the spring, the season when it is richest in this drying, styptic constituent.

The Ojibwa Indians pounded the inner bark of panicled dogwood and inserted the compressed mass into the anus to cure piles, while the Meskwakis recognized the astringent properties of wild black cherry, and injected a liquid solution of the boiled inner bark of this species into the rectum for the same purpose.

The Potawatomis employed an animal-bladder–bird-bone syringe to inject a tea of speckled alder bark, while the Menominees drank a bark tea of staghorn sumac to cure piles.

In the Southwest, the Zuni practitioner developed a unique method for treating bleeding piles. After inserting a moistened piece of rabbit skin into the rectum a few times, he dipped his moistened index finger into a dish of powdered cancer root and inserted it into the offended orifice, reputedly gaining quick, drying results.

INFLAMMATIONS AND SWELLINGS

ᥥᔦ WITCH HAZEL

Witch hazel was long utilized by the Indians before it was borrowed by the early settlers who soon adopted it into their own *materia medica*. Virgil J. Vogel carefully traced the history of this species, and it is from his account that I summarize the application of witch hazel in medicine.

The Menominees of Wisconsin boiled the leaves and rubbed the liquid on the legs of tribesmen who were participating in sporting games. This tribe apparently learned to prepare a witch hazel liniment from the Stockbridge Indians of Massachusetts when the latter group emigrated to Wisconsin. A decoction of the boiled twigs was used to cure aching backs, while steam derived by placing the twigs in water with hot rocks was a favorite Potawatomi treatment for muscular aches.

As early as 1744, it was observed that the Mohawks treated bruised eyes by applying a wash of steeped witch hazel bark. By 1850, the American Medical Association listed this plant as useful for treating piles, internal hemorrhages, and eye inflammations.

Witch hazel leaves were listed in the *U.S. Pharmacopoeia* from 1862 through 1916, and in the *National Formulary* from 1916 to 1955. They are generally used for relieving inflammation and bruises and for their astringent properties, on cuts, etc. As usual, it might be added, the *Dispensatory of the United States* is doubtful that witch hazel possesses any medicinal virtues.

The generic name, *Hamamelis*, is derived from two Greek words, *hama* and *melis*. The first word means "at the same time" and the second means "a fruit." This combination was chosen because witch hazel flowers appear in late fall at the same time its fruits of the previous year are ripening. The species name *Virginiana*, of course, refers to the locality of this species' cultivation, which at one time was in the southern states, especially in the low, damp woods of Virginia.

The popular name witch hazel was applied by those who once ascribed occult powers to this species and employed the forked branches as a divining rod in their searches for water and gold.

This indigenous shrub usually grows between eight and fifteen feet high, with a crooked stem covered with smooth brown bark. Aside from its oval, wavy-toothed leaves, its most peculiar characteristic is the fact that the bright yellow flowers appear in November or December, a time when most other trees and plants of its environment have generally lost their foliage. The large, shining black seeds which are ejected are edible. The Iroquois enjoyed a tea made of the boiled leaves sweetened with maple sugar as a warming, "natural" drink.

INFLUENZA

It would be foolish to imagine that the early Indians made a clear distinction between the symptoms of the common cold and the feverish, headachy, achy feelings of influenza. It is probable that the Indians utilized the same plants for colds as they did for influenza, namely, poplar buds, boneset, the wintergreens, wormwood, and the other species discussed under "Colds." Nevertheless, in this category are discussed those plants which seem to have been most frequently described by the Indians living in this century as being useful for the "flu." If the discussion on poison hemlock is too far from the thread of this book, the reader is invited to bypass this inclusion and skip on to the Indian remedies for "Insect Bites."

❧ HEMLOCK (FIG. 52)

The native evergreen forest hemlock is not to be confused with the poison hemlock of European origin. Whereas the former plant has been widely used in treating a variety of ills, the poisonous herb is best known for its role in the death of Socrates, as described by Plato. Before turning to this dangerous plant, the native medical uses of the "good" hemlocks will be described.

The Menominees prepared a tea of the hemlock inner bark and drank it to alleviate the symptoms of colds. A similar tea was used by the Forest Potawatomis to induce sweating and relieve colds and feverish conditions.

A related species, belonging to the yew family, was also used for influenzalike symptoms. The bark or twigs of ground hemlock was made into a tea by the Micmacs, the Penobscots, and other tribes. The Montagnais also used the twigs of this species, but they added club moss to the tea to treat the fever and loss of strength associated with influenzalike disorders.

Our physician-author of the last century, Dr. Millspaugh, aptly describes the uses to which hemlock was put in the late 1800s:

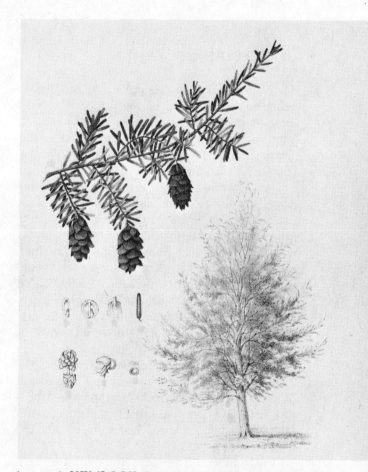

(FIG. 52) HEMLOCK: *Several tribes drank a tea of the inner bark of this evergreen to relieve influenzalike symptoms.*

A tired hunter arises fresh and invigorated from his bed of hemlock boughs, and the patient of the city physician, seeking health in our northern interiors, finds supreme comfort in a bath, in which hemlock leaves have been slowly steeping for some hours before his ablution, and quiet, refreshing slumber awaits him upon his couch of soft branches.

Hemlock pitch was official in the *U.S. Pharmacopoeia* from 1831 to 1894 when it was used externally as a gentle counterirritant for chronic rheumatic pains. Oil of hemlock, a derivative of this tree obtained by distilling the young branches, has been used in veterinary liniments.

The inner bark of the species of hemlock found in the west was used by the Indians of that region for bread. In an emergency the inner bark is edible in the raw, uncooked state. The Iroquois drank hemlock tea—this may be the Vitamin-C-rich drink that saved the first European "discoverers" of Canada from scurvy.

This typical Christmas card conifer attains a height of from sixty to eighty feet and is abundant in Canada and northern New England. It is also found in the mountainous regions of the central states, and a related species, western hemlock, extends to the Pacific coast. The leaves, or needles, appear flat or rounded at the tips as illustrated, and the top surfaces of hemlock needles are highly reflective, often showing the blueness of the sky. The small reddish brown cones dangle from the ends of the twigs and ripen in the fall.

The poison hemlock (FIG.53) was *not* utilized by the Indians of North America, but its fruits

(FIG. 53) *POISON HEMLOCK: This poisonous species was not used by the Indians of North America, but its fruits contain the deadly principle coniine which was formerly used in small quantities by American physicians as a pain-relieving drug. Poison hemlock, or conium, was responsible for the death of Socrates in Plato's* Phaedo.

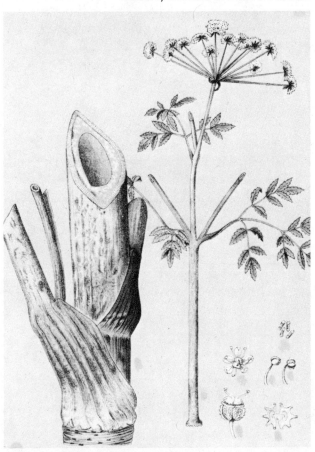

contain the deadly principle coniine which was formerly employed in small quantities by American physicians as an antispasmodic, a sedative, and a pain-relieving drug. It has since fallen into complete disuse.

Poison hemlock leaves resemble parsley leaves; for this reason, it is a doubly dangerous weed. Naturalized in this country from Europe, it has, often with fatal results, been mistaken for the common table herb. (See illustration.) It usually grows along roadsides or in waste places and attains a height of from two to five feet. Clusters of small, white flowers appear in June or July, and grayish green fruit appear in August. The whole plant has a fetid odor that has been compared to that of cat or mouse urine; it is especially noticeable when the plant is bruised. The poisonous properties vary according to temperature, soil, and climate, being most deadly in hot, dry weather and in tropical environments.

The alkaloid coniine is the most powerful of those contained within this plant. It effects paralysis of the peripheral endings of the motor nerves with only slight effects upon the nerves of sensation. Thus, Socrates' mind remained clear while his ability to use his muscles was gradually stolen from him by the deadly draught of conium. As Dr. Lawrence LeShan, the parapsychologist, has often said, he prefers to read the great authors to gain accurate descriptions of illnesses from the patients' own point of view. Thus, Tolstoy's account of stomach cancer in his *The Death of Ivan Ilyich* surpasses even the best "scientific" descriptions available. Similarly, Plato has so perfectly described in *Phaedo* the progress of conium poisoning in the death of Socrates that it is worth reading in its entirety.

Chinquapin is a low-growing shrub that belongs to the chestnut family. Its name, from the Algonquian, refers to the large, edible nuts. This species contains tannin and was used, like the chestnut tree, as an astringent in domestic American medicine. The nuts are nutritious, containing 45 percent starch and 2.5 percent protein. The Cherokees originally inhabited lands in the south where the Chinquapin grew in abundance. This great tribe treated influenzalike symptoms (sweating, headache, chills, fever) by applying a solution of the steeped leaves as an external wash on the patient.

INSECT BITES AND STINGS

Many plants were applied to insect stings and bites to alleviate the painful swelling; some of them are listed below. These have been selected to include at least one species from each geographical "Indian" division of North America, namely, the east, south, midwest, north central, southwest, and west.

FENDLER BLADDERPOD

The Navajos made a tea of the fendler bladderpod and used it as a remedy for the bites of spiders.

PURPLE CONEFLOWER

The Indians of the western plains used the purple coneflower as a universal application for the bites and stings of all crawling, flying, or leaping bugs. Between June and September, the bristly stemmed plant, which grows in dry open woods and on prairies, bears a striking purplish flower.

STIFF GOLDENROD

The Meskwaki Indians of the Minnesota region ground the flowers of the stiff goldenrod species into a lotion and applied it to bee stings. Many species of goldenrod were employed in Indian medicine, and the sweet-scented variety (*S. odora*) was on the secondary list of the *U.S. Pharmacopoeia* from 1820 to 1882, when it was employed for stimulant and diaphoretic purposes.

TRUMPET HONEYSUCKLE

The leaves of the trumpet honeysuckle species were ground by chewing and then applied to bee stings. This native plant is often cultivated, but in the wild state it is found growing on the borders of woods and thickets. It is a vine with leaves that are dark green above and white below. The trumpet-shaped flowers, which are bright red with yellowish interiors, bloom between April and September.

WILD ONION AND GARLIC (FIG.54)

To relieve the pain of insect stings the Dakotas and Winnebagos applied the crushed bulbs of wild onions and garlics. This genus has been used in folk medicine as well as by the Indians; the European species (A. *sativum*) was official in the pharmacopoeias of the United States and Britain when it was employed to rid the respiratory tract of phlegm, to rid the bowels of parasites, and to aid digestion.

(FIG. 54) WILD GARLIC: *To relieve the pain of insect stings, several tribes applied the crushed bulbs of wild onion and wild garlic.*

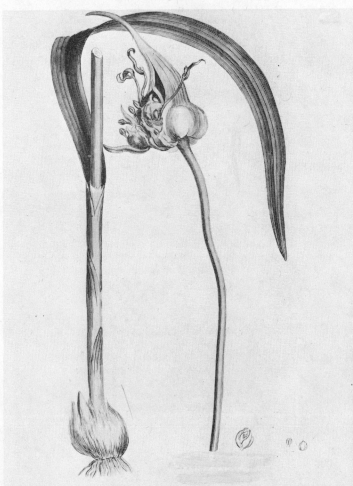

✖ PRICKLY PEAR

Although an Indian source is not listed, poultices of the prickly pear cactus were used in Texas as a home remedy for the bites of poisonous arthropods. (This genus is beautifully illustrated in "Warts.")

✖ SALTBUSH

The Navajos chewed the stems of the salt-bush and placed the pulpy mash on areas of swelling caused by the bites of ants, bees, and wasps. The Zuñis applied the dried, powdered roots and flowers mixed with saliva to ant bites. In the field, in an emergency, the fresh flowers were crushed and applied to stings and bites.

✖ SNAKEWEED

Another remedy of the Indians of the Southwest, snakeweed, was chewed by the Navajos and placed on the bites of bees, ants, and wasps.

✖ BROOM SNAKEWEED

Broom snakeweed, a shrubby plant, is found in the southwestern states and is especially abundant in northern Arizona. The Navajos chewed the stem and applied the resin to insect bites and stings of all kinds.

✖ WILD SUNFLOWER

The Hopi Indians applied the wild sunflower to spider bites.

✖ TOBACCO

Although tobacco is rapidly falling out of use, it was used widely in early medicine, both in Euorpe and America. A favority remedy for bee stings was the application of wet tobacco leaves. Many adventure stories tell us that explorers have often employed chewed tobacco leaves for the juice which is rubbed on the body as an insect repellent.

✖ WESTERN WOOD LILY

The Blackfoot treated the bite of a "small, brown, poisonous spider" with a wet dressing of the pulverized flowers of the western wood lily.

INSECT REPELLENTS AND INSECTICIDES

❧ CANADA FLEABANE (FIG.55)

The Cree Indians boiled Canada fleabane and drank the resulting tea to cure diarrhea; however, we learn from an early American herbalist, Samuel Stearns, that "the chief use of the *flea banes* is for destroying fleas and gnats, by burning the herbs so as to waste away in smoke."

The plant contains a volatile oil that is thought to act like oil of turpentine in the human system.

(FIG. 55) CANADA FLEABANE: *This common weed was burned and the smoke used to drive away fleas and gnats.*

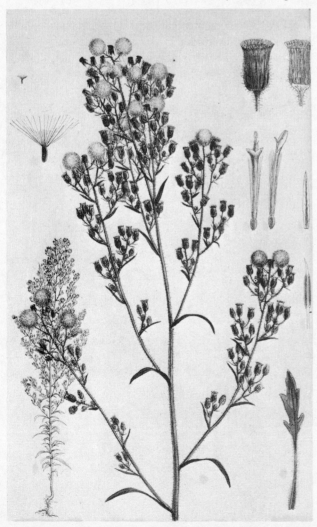

Probably because of the presence of this strong-smelling oil the plant was much used in Indian medicine. Aside from its employment to cure diarrhea, a tea made of the boiled root was taken for menstrual irregularities. To cure gonorrhea, the leaves were boiled and the resulting liquid applied externally; internally this liquid was used to treat hemorrhage. Tribes which have used this species in medicine include the Houmas, Ojibwas, Meskwakis, and the Catawbas.

Various species of fleabane have been official in the *U.S. Pharmacopoeia* when they were employed for their stimulant properties. The aromatic oil of erigeron has been used as a uterine stimulant and was official in the *U.S. Pharmacopoeia* from 1863 to 1916.

Fleabane is common throughout North America and is one of our gifts to Europe, where the weed has run wild and become naturalized. The height of this species varies from a few inches to ten feet, depending on the soil. The common features include hairy leaves and numerous heads of small, inconspicuous, white flowers which appear in North America from June to November.

❧ GOLDENSEAL (FIG.56)

The low perennial herb goldenseal was primarily employed for tonic, stimulant, and astringent purposes, first by the Indians and then by the early settlers. It is placed here as an insect repellent because the Cherokees seem to have favored this species for this purpose. Goldenseal could have been discussed under "Digestive Disorders" or "Inflammations" just as logically but is placed here to balance the text.

The Cherokees pounded the large rootstock with bear fat and smeared it on their bodies as an insect repellent. They also employed it as an internal remedy. In the Ohio River Valley it enjoyed some reputation as an astringent and was used for inflammation of the mucous membrane of the throat and for sore eyes. The root was also boiled in water and the resulting liquid applied as a wash for skin diseases, both by the Indians and in domestic American medicine. These diverse applications could be explained on the basis of the three alkaloids it contains, hydrastine, canadine, and berberine. The dried rootstock was official in the *U.S. Pharmacopoeia* from 1831 to 1842; it was readmitted in 1863 and remained

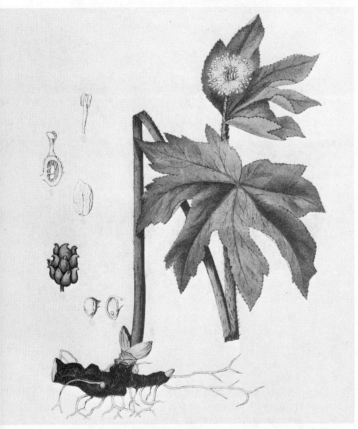

(FIG. 56) GOLDENSEAL: *This popular herb was used by the Cherokees, who pounded the large rootstock together with bear fat and smeared it on their bodies as an insect repellent.*

until 1936. Goldenseal is presently enjoying some popularity as a home remedy for stomach ailments and as a laxative.

Goldenseal was once abundant throughout the eastern United States and southeastern Canada but is now almost extinct due to overcollection by short-sighted herb dealers. Goldenseal root was bringing from $1.00 to $1.50 a pound in 1909 when other, more easily found, medicinal plants brought wholesale prices of from 2½ to 5 cents a pound. When used for medicines, the yellow rootstock was dug in the autumn after the plant had withered.

Besides being used to repel insects, for sore eyes, and for digestive disorders, goldenseal was used by many tribes as a yellow dye to color their clothing and implements of warfare.

To protect potato plants from insects, the Menominee Indians boiled the May apple plant and splashed the resulting liquid on their potato crops. The Indians of Mendocino County, California, crushed California laurel leaves and spread them about their lodgings to repel fleas. A natural insecticide was derived by burning the powdered leaves of Texas croton, the smoke driving away all flying and crawling pests. In the Northwest the Blackfoot Indians prepared an insect repellent from the dried flowers of the pineapple weed. Juniper berries have been crushed and the oil rubbed on the skin as an insect repellent, while some Indians used the root juice of bloodroot, or puccoon, in the same way.

It has recently been determined that rotenone, a natural insecticide, is present in devil's shoe-string. This species was used by some tribes to destroy intestinal worms. Various rotenone-containing plants have been used as fish poisons in South America and the East Indies for centuries. This natural insecticide is especially effective against flying insects and appears to be relatively harmless to mammals.

Before leaving the insect repellents, we must return to tobacco leaves. Nicotine was once used on a large scale to eliminate crop pests, and although it was an effective agent, it has largely been replaced by synthetic organic insecticides, namely DDT (chlorophenothane). Although tobacco leaves were used by some Indians of South America to repel insects, the North American tribes did not use them in that way. It will be interesting to see whether ground tobacco leaves will again be used as an insecticide now that DDT has proved to be more dangerous than beneficial.

INSOMNIA

✤§ PARTRIDGEBERRY

Although partridgeberry plant was utilized by the Indians primarily to facilitate childbirth, the Menominees drank a tea made of the steeped leaves to cure insomnia.

This evergreen creeper contains a bitter principle and tannin, a tissue-drying agent. It was official in the *National Formulary* from 1926 to 1947 when it was used as an astringent, a tonic, and a diuretic.

✤§ BLACK NIGHTSHADE (FIG.57)

An annual herb, the black nightshade grows in Europe, the United States, South America, and in some Pacific islands. Although its country of origin has not been finally determined, it was collected on the Columbia River at Baker's Bay as early as 1825.

It is not known whether the Indians learned to use nightshade on their own, but this species has been used in medicine, especially for inflammations, from the time of Dioscorides (A.D. 54). The bruised leaves were applied to burns in Arabic medicine, while in other countries the plant has been used to produce sleep.

In North America, it is reported that the Comanches, Houmas, and Rappahannock Indians used nightshade to treat tuberculosis, to expel worms, and to cure sleeplessness, respectively. The last-named tribe prepared their remedy for insomnia by steeping a small amount of the leaves in a large quantity of water.

Although some authorities claim the fruits are safe to eat, citing the fact that in the Dakotas the berries are cultivated on a large scale as a substitute for blueberries, others state that the berries have sometimes proved harmful to some people and that a fatal case of poisoning in a child who ate the unripe fruit was reported in 1901. How can the berries be used for pies and preserves by some and prove harmful, even fatal, to others? The *Dispensatory of the United States* offers a clue.

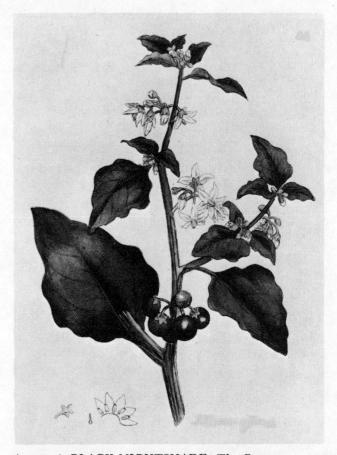

(FIG. 57) BLACK NIGHTSHADE: *The Rappahannock Indians of Virginia drank a tea made of the leaves of this herb as a remedy for insomnia.*

"It is probably that the proportion of *solanine* is less in the ripe berries than in the unripe and it may be that some of the toxicity is destroyed in the process of cooking."

In any case, this species is not to be confused with deadly nightshade, or belladonna (FIG.58), from which the powerful drug atropine is derived. Belladonna is a combination of two Italian words, *bella*, or "beautiful," and *donna*, or "lady." Some writers believe that the berries of this species were used by Italian ladies as a cosmetic dye and as a dilator of the eye pupil to give them a captivating look.

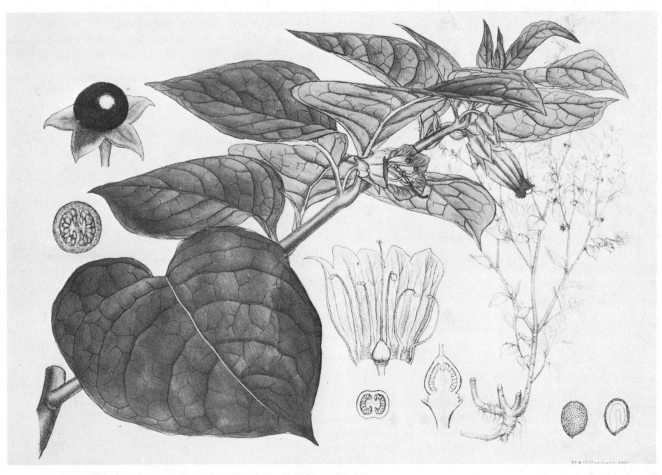

(FIG. 58) *DEADLY NIGHTSHADE (BELLADONNA): The powerful drug atropine is derived from this plant.*

Unscrupulous or ignorant drug collectors have so frequently substituted the leaves of the black nightshade for belladonna leaves that earlier works on medicinal plants exhibited photographs of microscopic details of both species to alert wholesale drug dealers.

✃ LADY'S-SLIPPER (FIG.59)

The lady's-slipper was first used by several tribes as a sedative and nerve medicine; it later became accepted in domestic American medicine as a cure for insomnia. Rafinesque, a medical-botanist of the first half of the nineteenth century, introduced this plant to medical circles.

Of this beautiful genus, all the species are equally medical; they have been long known to the Indians. . . . They are sedative, nervine, antispasmodic, etc. . . . They produce beneficial effects in all nervous diseases and hysterical affections, by allaying pain, quieting the nerves and promoting sleep. They are also used in . . . epilepsy, tremors, nervous fever, etc., . . . having no baneful nor narcotic effects. The dose is a teaspoonful of the powder (root), diluted in sugar-water, or any other convenient form.

Root decoctions were used for "female problems" by the Menominees and the Pillager Ojibwas. The Penobscots prepared a tea of a related species and drank it to calm the nerves.

Lady's-slipper appears to be another drug plant that was once popularly prescribed in medicine but has since been superseded by synthetic agents. During the time the roots were official in the U.S. *Pharmacopoeia*, from 1863 to 1916, they were primarily employed as an antispasmodic and as a nerve medicine. As Dr. Millspaugh stated in 1878:

Cypripedium acts as a sedative to the nerves in general, causing a sense of mental quiet and lassitude, and subduing nervous and mental irritation. It seems also to quiet spasms of voluntary muscles, and hysterical attacks, especially in women. This is one of our drugs that has not been sufficiently thought of by provers. It merits a full proving. . . .

And the plant remains "unproved" to this day!

This beautiful member of the orchid family is found in bogs and wet places from Nova Scotia to Nebraska, south to Mississippi and Alabama. The plant has an erect stem that grows between one and two feet in height. Its leaves are large, elliptic to oval, with parallel veins; they contain hairs which cause a rash similar to that of poison ivy in some people. The plant bears a single, yellow, terminal flower between May and June. When gathered for use in medicine, the rhizome and roots were dug in the fall, cleaned in water, and dried in the shade.

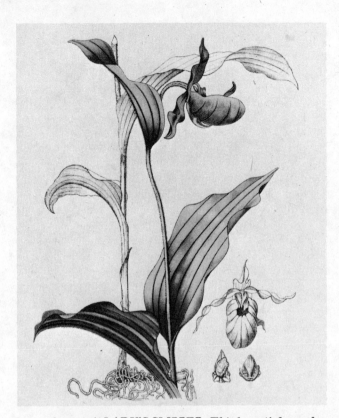

(FIG. 59) LADY'S-SLIPPER: *This beautiful member of the orchid family was first used by several tribes as a sedative and nerve medicine and later became accepted in domestic American medicine as a cure for insomnia.*

KIDNEY AND BLADDER AILMENTS

The native American recognized that swollen extremities sometimes resulted from a failing heart or weak kidneys. He used many different applications on the affected arm or leg in an attempt to encourage the outflow of this excess fluid in the form of urine. Diuretic drugs, when effective, increase the rate of urine flow; the Navajos evidently recognized this because one of their favorite plant remedies was called "urine spurter."

✺ BEARBERRY (FIG. 60)

The Thompson Indians of British Columbia drank a tea of the steeped leaves of bearberry to promote the flow of urine and to strengthen the

(FIG. 60) BEARBERRY: *The Thompson Indians of British Columbia drank a tea of the steeped leaves to promote the flow of urine and to strengthen the bladder and kidneys.*

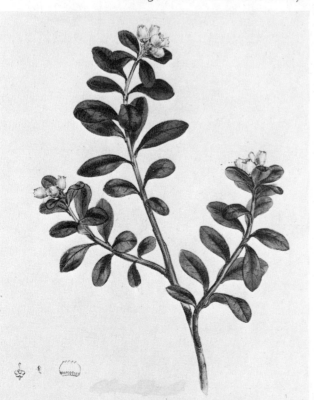

bladder and kidneys; the Menominees added the leaves to remedies associated with women's disorders. It appears as though the bearberry was discovered independently, by both the Indian and by his white counterpart. Although this evergreen shrub had been used in ancient medicine, it was not popularly employed for kidney disorders until the middle of the eighteenth century.

From this time on, the bearberry leaf was recognized for its diuretic properties; it was admitted to the *London Pharmacopoeia* in 1763 and the *U.S. Pharmacopoeia* in 1820, where it remained until 1936.

Bearberry is indigenous to Europe, Asia, the United States, and Canada. It grows in dry, sandy, or rocky soil and appears as a low, branching shrub with thick, leathery leaves and waxy whitish flowers. The smooth, red fruits, about the size of a pea, are very prominent from August to late winter. The edible berries are favored by bear and grouse, and the dried leaves were formerly mixed with tobacco, forming an Indian smoking mixture known as *sagack-homi* in Canada, and *kinikinik* among the western American tribes.

✺ MILKWEED

The Natchez Indians, originally from the southern Mississippi region, treated kidney problems by drinking a root tea made of milkweed three times a day. The patient was advised to avoid salty foods.

To treat kidney ailments in their part of the continent, the Blackfoot Indians soaked the seeds of Rocky Mountain juniper and drank the resulting tea. They also utilized a tea made by boiling the roots of Wild Black Currant. The Potawatomis of the prairies boiled the green fruits of dogbane, while the Flambeau Ojibwas used a tea made of the roots and stems to cleanse the kidneys of pregnant women.

Other plants used as diuretics include the pounded roots of button snakeroot, a favorite Creek remedy; sarsaparilla, a favorite of the Plains tribes; and the wintergreens, once popular among the Dakotas and the Winnebagos.

LAXATIVES

CASCARA SAGRADA

Of all plant medicines of the North American Indians, cascara sagrada is presently the best known, and an extract of the bark is frequently prescribed for its laxative effects. This tree is native to the northwest Pacific Coast and ranges from southern British Columbia to California. It was utilized for its laxative effects throughout its range by various tribes, and several varieties are known which exert similar effects.

It was most probably from the Indians of Mendocino County that the early Spanish priests of California learned of this "sacred bark," as they named it. In 1877, Dr. J. H. Bundy rediscovered this drug plant, probably through the Indians; through him it was introduced into medicine and rapidly became a favorite laxative throughout the world. In 1890, cascara bark was admitted to the *U.S. Pharmacopoeia* where today a fluid extract of it is still an official medicine. It is marketed in various forms and is known as Danthron, Sennapod, Senekot, Cassanthranol, and Peri-Colase.

Cascara sagrada is employed to treat habitual constipation; it acts by irritating the bowel and inducing peristalsis. The *Dispensatory of the United States* adds that "it often appears to restore tone to the relaxed bowel and in this way produce a permanent beneficial effect."

The Thompson Indians of British Columbia prepared a laxative drink by boiling a small amount of the bark or wood in water. This was a standard method of preparing plant medicines and consistently reappears throughout the literature on Indian remedies.

This native tree is common to the base and sides of canyons throughout its Pacific range. It is a small tree, seldom higher than fifteen to twenty feet, and has dark green elliptical leaves that are from two to six inches long. It bears small, greenish flowers which are followed by black berries. When collected for medicine, the bark is stripped from the trunk in the spring and summer and carefully dried. It is then aged for several years before being used, one year from the time of gathering being a minimum for this aging process.

Indiscriminate cutting has destroyed great stands of these trees, and as early as 1909 Alice Henkel wrote about this problem:

> Many trees are annually destroyed in the collection of cascara sagrada, as they are usually peeled to such an extent that no new bark is formed. It has been estimated that one tree furnishes approximately 10 pounds of bark, and granting a crop of 1,000,000 pounds a year, 100,000 trees are thus annually destroyed. . . .

This destructive attitude towards a useful species is far removed from that of the Hopi who looks upon all living things as an extension of himself. As Whiting has shown:

> When a Hopi man goes out to gather some kind of plant of which he finds himself in need, he does not fail to carry the proper kind of prayer offering with him. When he sees the plant, he places this offering beside it but does not pick this particular one for it will carry the message of his need to the other plant people. Instead he goes on until he finds other plants of the same kind which he will gather.

AMERICAN SENNA (FIG. 61)

American senna is, like the senna of European origin, widely employed for its laxative properties. The Indians were aware of this plant, and they employed it in a variety of ways; not one of them, however, indicated that they recognized it as a laxative. The Cherokees applied the root, pounded with water, to sores; they drank a decoction of it to reduce fevers. Other tribes utilized wild senna (another of its common names) to ease sore throat.

The leaves of the senna were widely used for their cathartic properties and were official in the

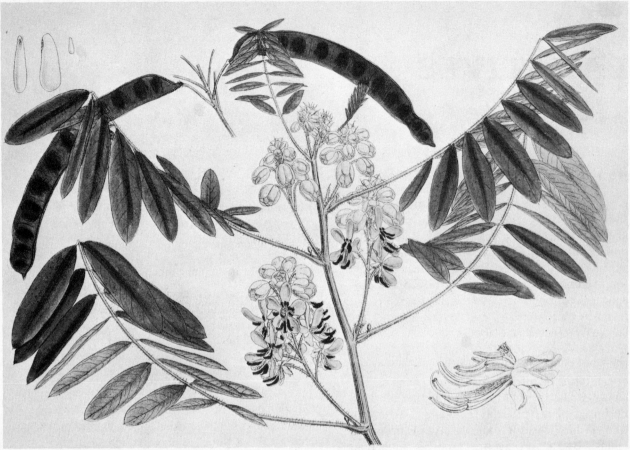

(FIG. 61) AMERICAN SENNA: *The leaves of this plant are widely used for their laxative properties.*

U.S. *Pharmacopoeia* from 1820 to 1882. They were gathered at the time of flowering, which is during July or August.

American senna is found in wet soil in the eastern and central United States and Canada. Its leaves appear as they do in the illustration, and the numerous flowers which appear from August to September are yellow in color and are borne on slender, fuzzy stems.

⊷§ MAY APPLE (FIG.62)

The Indians used the root of the May apple for its cathartic effects long before it was rediscovered and borrowed for American medicine. Although the drug is described as a "drastic purgative," or cathartic, it is well to remember that an early visitor to North America reported that an Indian woman had used the root to commit suicide. In another case, this one verified in a medical journal in 1890, a sixty-year-old woman died after ingesting five grams of the resin. Nevertheless, as is so with many poisonous substances, in smaller quantities the May apple is used as a

(FIG. 62) MAY APPLE: *Although poisonous in large dosage, in smaller quantities the roots were used for their laxative effects by the Indians long before the plant was rediscovered and borrowed for American medicine.*

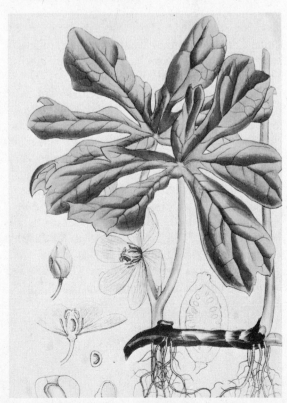

medicine. To cure chronic constipation it is sometimes mixed with cascara sagrada.

✸ BUSH BEANS

To induce bowel movement, the Penobscots chewed bush beans.

✸ BUTTERNUT

The butternut is discussed and illustrated in "Digestive Disorders." It became official in the *U.S. Pharmacopoeia* in 1820, and was one of the most popular naturally occurring laxatives of the last century.

✸ BLUE FLAG

The Creeks employed the rhizome of the blue flag to such an extent that it was cultivated by them in each of their villages. It was later adopted by American physicians and was long used in medicine for its cathartic properties. (This species is treated in greater detail under "Wounds.")

✸ AMERICAN IPECAC (FIG.63)

The following tribes all used the root of the ipecac (in small doses) to encourage bowel

(FIG. 63) IPECAC: *Several diverse tribes used the root of this native species to encourage bowel movements.*

movements or (in larger doses) to induce vomiting: the Creeks, Apaches, Ojibwas, and the Meskwakis. In general, the roots were eaten raw.

Whereas the Indians looked upon vomiting as a cleansing act, this action of American ipecac too often accompanied its laxative effects and it was eventually dropped from medical practice, being replaced by less powerful drugs, namely senna and cascara sagrada.

✸ CULVER'S ROOT (FIG.64)

The early settlers quickly learned the value of Culver's root from the Indians. The Senecas made a tea of the root and drank it as a laxative, while the Menominees and Meskwakis used it for this and other medicinal purposes.

The roots were gathered in the fall and stored for at least one year before being used. This is another plant that was accepted in the *U.S. Pharmacopoeia* for its laxative effects; however, it was eventually dropped as being too drastic and irregular in its action.

(FIG. 64) CULVER'S ROOT: *The early settlers learned from the Seneca Indians to make a laxative tea of the roots of this plant.*

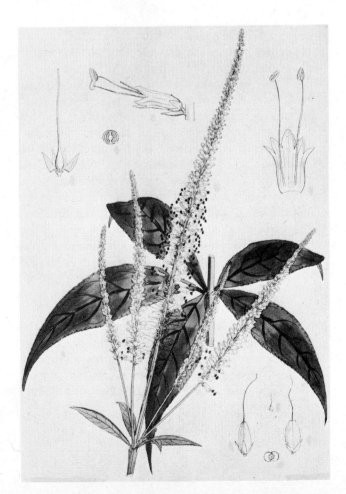

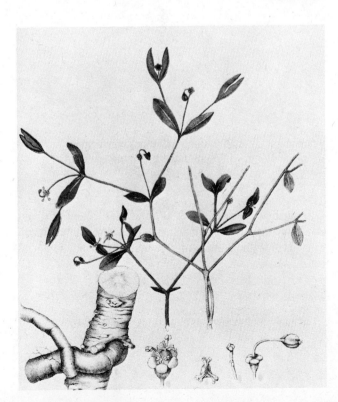

MEASLES

Archeological evidence indicates that measles was unknown among the American Indians prior to the arrival of the European. Instances are recorded of total decimation of a tribe following contact with an infected traveler. As might be expected, the Indian employed the following botanical remedies to treat the high fever associated with the disease rather than to destroy the causative organism, which was then unknown.

৯৪ LICORICE FERN

The licorice fern was employed in the treatment of measles by the Cowlitz Indians of Washington, who prepared a tea of the pounded, boiled rhizome mixed with fir needles. This tribe also treated coughs by chewing and slowly swallowing the juice of the roasted rhizome.

৯৪ SASSAFRAS (FIG.65)

To lower fever and to promote the eruption of the rash in measles, the Rappahannock tribe of Virginia drank an infusion of sassafras roots. This remedy was also employed by the Houmas. Most Indian tribes of the eastern United States utilized this plant for one ailment or another.

Sassafras became one of the most important articles of export early in the history of the nation, the bulk of the shipments going to England for use in treating colic, venereal disease, pain, etc. The tree is a native of North America and was first discovered (after the Indians) by the Spaniards when they conquered Florida in 1538. These Europeans mistook the scent of sassafras for cinnamon, a spice which grows in Ceylon. Around 1560, sassafras was brought to Spain, where it soon acquired a great reputation for curing various diseases.

Sassafras has been an important "tonic" in domestic medicine. Rural general practitioners were especially fond of sassafras tea for treating high blood pressure and for promoting perspiration in colds. The Pennsylvania Germans used the flowers in a tea to reduce fevers and the berries as a wine for colds.

Derivatives of this tree are still widely used in a number of commerical products. The aromatic

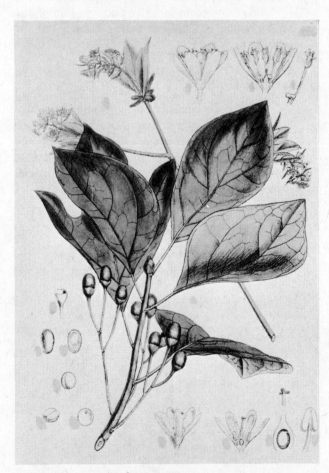

(FIG. 65) *SASSAFRAS: To lower fever and to promote the eruption of the rash in measles, the Rappahannock tribe of Virginia drank a tea made from sassafras roots.*

oil, safrole, is used as an antiseptic agent in dentistry, as a flavoring agent, and as an ingredient in root beer, chewing gum, toothpaste, and mouthwashes.

The root bark was official in the *U.S. Pharmacopoeia* from 1820 through 1926 when its volatile oil, also safrole, was used as a pain reliever.

This native tree is found in thickly wooded areas from Maine to Ontario and south to Florida and Texas. In the North it occurs as a shrub while it may grow upwards of one hundred feet in the South. The bark is gray and ridged irregularly, and the leaves vary considerably in outline—from oval to mitten-shaped. The blossoms appear in April or May, are yellowish green in color, and are aromatic. The dark blue fruits, which ripen in September, are borne on a thick, red stalk and are about the size of a pea.

MENSTRUATION

The Indians employed plant remedies for three categories of menstrual problems. There were preparations to encourage delayed menstruation, to reduce profuse menstruation, and to relieve cramps and pain. During their "periods," women usually lived apart from their families in a separate facility. Taboos restricted their actions so that among the Cherokees we read an account where a decoction of skullcap was "used as a wash to counteract the ill effects of eating food prepared by a woman in the menstrual condition, or when such a woman by chance comes into a sick room. . . ." (As a side note, women of the Ankara tribe made "sanitary napkins" from pieces of buffalo skin that had been smoked.)

To encourage delayed menstruation, several species of wild carrot were used in many different ways by several tribes; however, none reportedly employed it as a menstrual excitant for which purpose it was official in the *U.S. Pharmacopoeia* from 1820 to 1882. One clinical experiment has shown that extracts of wild carrot can induce uterine contraction.

⤳ WHITE CEDAR (ARBORVITAE)
(FIG. 66)

Menominee women drank a tea of steeped inner white cedar bark to promote menstruation. Other Indian tribes used white cedar to relieve headache and heart pain and to reduce swellings. The leaves yield *oil of white cedar,* which is used internally to promote menstruation and to relieve rheumatism. This volatile oil is toxic, and poisoning from overdoses has frequently occurred. The action of this oil is similar to that of camphor, stimulating the heart and causing convulsions in high dosage. The twigs of arborvitae were official in the *U.S. Pharmacopoeia* from 1882 to 1894 when they were used to promote menstruation, as a stimulant, and for diuretic purposes.

In *The Original Journals of Lewis and Clark,* the use of arborvitae wood by the Indians to manufacture bows, baskets, canoes, hats, cord, and

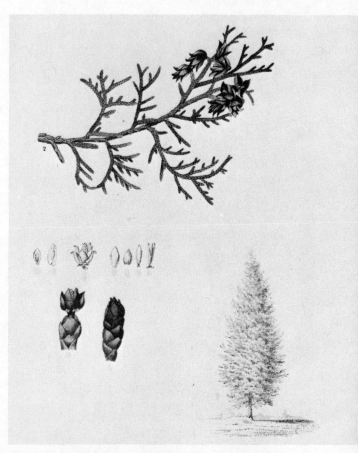

(FIG. 66) ARBORVITAE: *To promote menstruation, Menominee women drank a tea made from the inner bark of this tall conifer.*

roofing is described. Since this soft, light wood also resists decay, it is used for fence posts, shingles, and telephone poles.

This conifer attains a height of seventy feet and grows in swampy areas and along stream banks from New Brunswick to Manitoba and south to Illinois and North Carolina, often in impenetrable forests, or "cedar swamps." The old bark appears in irregular strips while the wood is reddish in color, soft, and fine grained. Its cones are four to six inches long, and the seeds have broad wings. The twigs are covered by tight-fitting scales that have a reptilelike quality. The arborvitae appears as a solid, yellowish green column throughout our northern forests.

BLACK COHOSH (FIG.67)

One of the Indian uses for the black cohosh was to treat "women's problems," which would explain why it was also known as squawroot. Between 1820 and 1936, when the plant was official in the *U.S. Pharmacopoeia*, the rhizome and

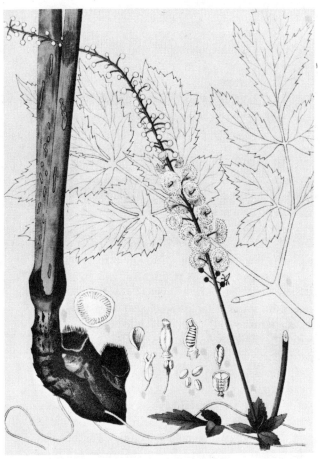

(FIG. 67) *BLACK COHOSH: One of the Indian uses for this plant was for treating "women's problems," which would explain why it was also known as squawroot. It was once an official drug in the* United States Pharmacopoeia, *where it was listed as a sedative, a medication for rheumatism, and a medication to promote menstruation.*

roots were used in the United States as a sedative, for rheumatism, and to promote menstruation. This species is easily recognized during the summer when its slender, candlelike flowers rise in clusters of from one to three feet in length, thus standing above most of the other woodland flowers. Black cohosh grows throughout eastern North America, while most of the commerical supply was collected in September, after the fruit had ripened, in the Blue Ridge Mountains. The flowers emit a very unpleasant odor, which was thought to repel insects. This explains another of its common names—bugbane, or bugwort. This insect-repelling quality was apparent to the botanist Linnaeus because the generic name, *Cimicifuga*, means in Latin "to drive away bugs." The specific name, *racemosa*, refers to the clustered grouping of its flowers.

SKULLCAP (FIG.68)

The Cherokees drank an infusion of the indigenous herb skullcap to promote suppressed menstruation.

Whether this usage was known before Dr. Van Derveer undertook his experiments with this species in 1772 is unknown. In any case, this Indian medicinal species was reported to be effective in the treatment of rabies, and soon the word spread; people began using it as an antihydrophobic, and it became popularly known as mad dog skullcap.

Dr. Millspaugh points out that the family to

(FIG. 68) SKULLCAP: *To promote retarded menstruation, the Cherokees drank a tea made from this interesting herb.*

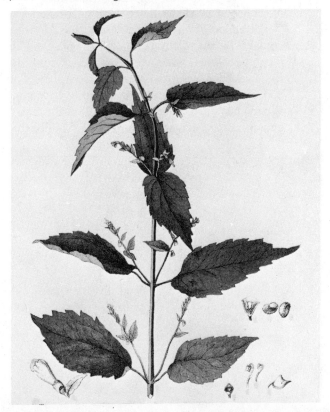

which this species belongs "yields many species . . . that are valued by the aborigines of countries in which they grow as antihydrophobics." He then reminded his pharmacologist colleagues to experiment with skullcap, "as native medication is always the result of long and more or less successful experiment."

Skullcap was accepted into medical circles in 1863 when the dried herb was entered in the *U.S. Pharmacopoeia*. There it remained until 1916 when it was removed and shifted to the *National Formulary*. The plant was employed for sedative and antispasmodic purposes so it is possible that mad dog skullcap may have been of some real value as originally stated in 1772.

❧ TANSY

Already described for its uses as an abortifacient, tansy leaf tea was also used by the Catawba Indians to promote menstruation. It has long been used in Europe as a bitter tea for its tonic properties and was then recommended "in the hysteria, especially when this disease is supposed to proceed from menstrual obstructions."

The leaves and flowering tops contain resins, camphor, borneol, and thujone. It has been internally used in domestic medicine to destroy intestinal worms and externally to kill fleas and lice.

The yellow flowers grow in clusters and bloom from July to September. Tansy grows from eighteen to forty inches tall along roadsides from Nova Scotia to Missouri and North Carolina.

To reduce profuse menstruation, several tribes employed a tea of the roots of blue cohosh. This plant was best known as a parturient, and the Indians called it squawroot or papoose root. The plant is a perennial herb that is said to have antispasmodic and diuretic properties. It is illustrated and discussed in greater detail under "Childbirth."

To relieve cramps and pain associated with menstruation, the Rappahannock Indians of Virginia drank a tea made of pennyroyal leaves or of spicebush twigs. For the same purpose, Kiowa women boiled the blossoms of dandelion with pennyroyal leaves and drank the resulting tea. Both pennyroyal and dandelion are discussed elsewhere in this book.

❧ SPICEBUSH

The native species spicebush was first employed in Indian medicine and later integrated into the homes and medical practice of the settlers. It was especially well known for its aromatic buds, bark, and berries. During the Revolutionary War, the Americans used the powdered berries as a substitute for allspice. The leaves were sometimes brewed in place of tea. In domestic medicine the plant was used to induce sweating and to reduce fever. The oil was often rubbed on the body to relieve rheumatic pains. At the beginning of this century, the bark was used as a remedy against worms.

This shrub belongs to the aromatic laurel family, which also gives us camphor and cinnamon. . Our native plant, the uses of which are described above, is closely related to the "official" benzoin, a tree that grows in southeastern Asia. This plant yields the balsamic resin benzoin, which is described as an antiseptic, a stimulant, a diuretic, and an expectorant.

It appears as if our native species, the one used by Rappahannock women to allay the pain and cramps that are sometimes associated with menstruation, also contains benzoin. Both the native and the Asian plants yield a gummy balsam. Interestingly, this aromatic gum is burnt by some Hindus as an incense in their temples.

MILK SECRETION

The Indians universally practiced nursing an infant until it was three or four years old, while such foods as blueberries and prechewed meat slowly added to the baby's diet. One tribe of the Southwest, the Arikaras, substituted a mash of ground corn and buffalo meat in water when there was an insufficient flow of mother's milk. Many different plants were used to induce the secretion of milk, a few of which follow.

↝ WHITE BANEBERRY (FIG.69)

For the same purposes as above, Cheyenne women drank an infusion of the leaves of the white baneberry. It is easily distinguished by its oval-shaped snow-white berries, which are tipped with purple and stand on thick red stalks.

↝ TALL BLUE LETTUCE

The Ojibwas boiled the leaves of tall blue lettuce, and their women drank the resulting tea to relieve plugged milk ducts. The same preparation but using a related species, prickly lettuce, was taken by Meskwaki women to promote the secretion of milk.

↝ SPURGE (FIG.70)

The Zuñis were probably aware of the dangerous properties of plants belonging to the toxic

(FIG. 69) WHITE BANEBERRY: *To encourage the flow of milk in nursing women, the Cheyenne drank a tea made of the leaves of this colorful herb.*

(FIG. 70) SPURGE: *To promote the secretion of milk, Zuñi women drank a concoction of "four pinches" of this dangerous plant in one cup of warm white cornmeal mash.*

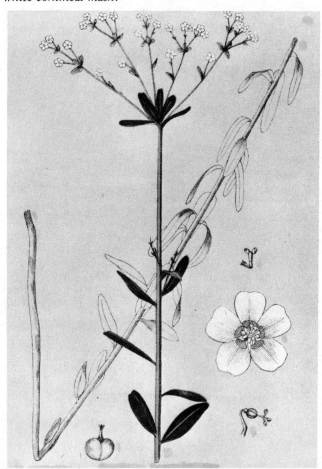

spurge family. One of their recipes, which was used to promote the flow of milk, calls for only "four pinches" of the pulverized spurge plant in one cup of warm white cornmeal mash. The species illustrated, the flowering spurge, was used by the Indians to cleanse the bowels. The milky juice that flows from the bruised plant was sometimes used as a vesicant to promote blistering in various infected conditions.

ᴥ§ SKELETON WEED

The skeleton weed was one of the most widely used lactagogue, or milk-inducing, plants. The Pawnee, Ponca, Omaha, and Blackfoot tribes utilized a tea of the steeped leaves to increase the flow of milk in nursing mothers, while the Cheyenne thought so highly of this species that they named it milk medicine. There are no records which indicate that this plant was employed in domestic or "official" medicine; nevertheless, the frequency with which the skeleton weed was used by various Indian tribes to stimulate the secretion of milk very definitely makes this a promising plant.

This perennial herb is common to the plains from Minnesota to Saskatchewan, Montana, Wisconsin, Missouri, Nebraska, Kansas, and Arizona. It is composed of a thick woody root, narrow lance-like upper leaves, with wider, lower leaves, and it grows between eight and eighteen inches high. The flower heads are three to four inches broad and usually bear five flowers.

Another species that was employed in cases of insufficient milk secretion is the eastern bracken fern. The rhizome was pounded and steeped in water and then drunk by Menominee women to relieve plugged milk ducts. The rhizome of this species was an important food item in New Zealand among the Maoris, and the boiled fronds are still eaten in Japan.

The Hopi Indians reportedly utilized the bedstraw milkweed to increase the flow of milk; however, the specific part used and the method of preparation are not known.

MOUTH SORES

❧ EUROPEAN BARBERRY

The roots of the introduced European barberry were pulverized in a little water and applied to mouth ulcers by the Penobscots of Maine, while the Catawba tribe drank a tea of the boiled roots and stems for stomach ulcers.

The fruits of this shrub were formerly used in England to reduce fevers, while the bark was employed as a purgative and as a diarrhea treatment. During the early part of the nineteenth century, the acidic berries were also used in Egypt to reduce fevers.

❧ GOLDTHREAD (FIG.71)

Both the Indians and early white settlers used the small goldthread root as a remedy for sore and ulcerated mouths. Interestingly, there is a consistency in this usage among many tribes. The Mohegans boiled the root in water as a mild gargle for mouth sores; the Montagnais used the same preparation to rinse mouth sores; and the Penobscot tribe chewed the stems to retard sores in the mouth. Similar use of goldthread was made by the Menominees, the Potawatomis, and the Pillager Ojibwas.

Goldthread contains the alkaloid berberine, which has mild sedative action, and the plant has been widely used as a folk remedy in treating inflammations of the mucous membrane of the mouth or eyes.

This attractive, small member of the crowfoot family commonly occurs in dark swamps and dense forests. It is most prevalent in northern New York, Michigan, the New England states, and Canada, but it is also found from Alaska south to Maryland. It is a small plant, only three to six inches high, and its threadlike gold roots grow near to the surface of the ground. The ever-

(FIG. 71) GOLDTHREAD: *Both the Indians and the early white settlers used this small root as a remedy for sore and ulcerated mouth.*

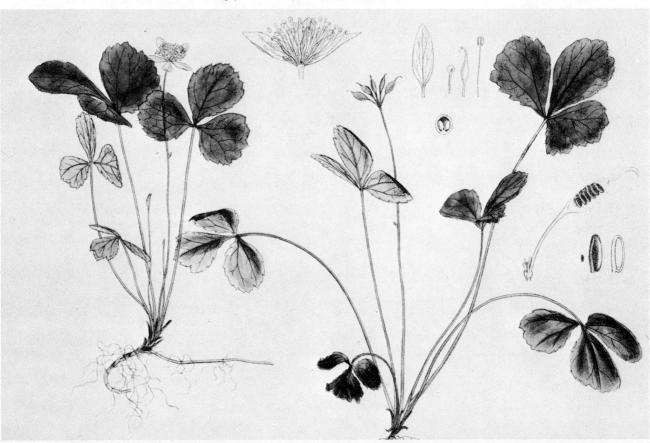

green leaves are three-lobed and glisten on the upper surface. The solitary, white, star-shaped flower is borne on the end of a stalk and has five to six petallike sepals appearing from May to July.

Autumn was the preferred time for collecting goldthread roots. The surrounding ground vegetation was discarded, and the tiny roots dried for market where in 1908 they brought from sixty to seventy cents a pound.

Goldthread was official in the *U.S. Pharmacopoeia* from 1820 to 1882 and in the *National Formulary* from 1916 to 1936, when it was employed as a bitter tonic and for treating inflammations of the mucous membranes of the mouth or eyes.

◦§ WILD PLUM

The Meskwakis boiled the scraped inner bark of wild plum and gargled the resulting solution to cure mouth sores. This native species is found from Connecticut to Montana and Colorado, south to Florida and Texas. It rarely exceeds thirty-five feet in height and bears red or yellow fruits from August to October.

◦§ SMOOTH UPLAND SUMAC

The root of smooth upland sumac was chewed fresh as a cure for sores in the mouth by Indians of British Columbia and was widely used in medicines by other American Indians. This species is discussed further under other topics (see index).

There were many other treatments for mouth ulcers; several of them are listed below. The Kiowas extracted the juice of the berries of red cedar by chewing and held the liquid in their mouths as a mild antiseptic rinse. The Catawba Indians boiled yellow root and utilized the liquid as a rinse, while the Indians of California infrequently employed the common horsetail fern for the same purpose. The whole plant was dried and fired on hot coals, and the ashes then applied to the mouth sores.

MOUTHWASH

✑ GERANIUM

Geranium roots were steeped in water and employed as a rinse for pyorrhea and inflamed gums by the Meskwaki tribe. The rhizome of this perennial herb was formerly collected in September or October and used in domestic medicine as an astringent because of its tannin content.

(FIG. 72) PEPPERMINT: *The fresh leaves of peppermint make an excellent mouthwash, leaving an agreeable taste after an initial sensation of heat.*

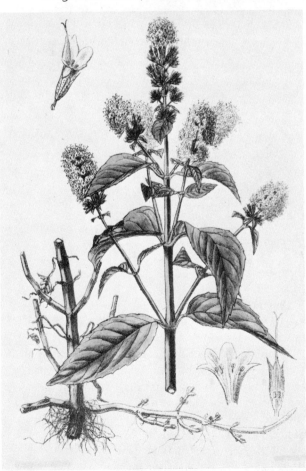

✑ PEPPERMINT (FIG. 72)

There is only one tribe reported as having used peppermint leaves. The Menominees treated pneumonia with a tea of peppermint, catnip, and American wild mint leaves. Nevertheless, peppermint leaves are widely used for flavoring candies, liqueurs, and chewing gums. The fresh leaves make an excellent mouthwash, leaving an agreeable taste after an initial sensation of heat. Menthol, the principal constituent of peppermint oil, is responsible for imparting the pleasant flavor. Peppermint oil is used medicinally as an agent to remove an excess of gases from the stomach and intestines and as a stimulant.

The genus name, *Mentha*, has its origins in Greek mythology where the nymph Mintha was supposedly metamorphosed into the form of this plant. The Latin word *piper* alludes to the aromatic qualities assigned to this species, thus named *piperita*.

Peppermint is a perennial herb naturalized from Europe, where it was frequent in regions of low, damp soils. It is now found growing wild in the eastern United States and is extensively cultivated in Michigan, Oregon, and New York.

✑ YERBA SANTA

Yerba santa was the most highly valued medicinal plant among the Indians of Mendocino County, California. The leaves were smoked and chewed like tobacco to treat asthma, or taken as a tea for colds. A natural mouthwash was prepared by rolling the leaves into balls and then allowing them to dry in the sun. The resulting spherical lumps were said to taste bitter at first, when chewed, but this was followed by a cool, sweet sensation if the user soon took a drink of water. As one Indian of this region put it, "It makes one taste kind of sweety inside."

MUMPS

The viral disease of mumps was little understood by the American Indian. It was probably nonexistent on this continent until the coming of the European, and as happened with so many other "new" diseases, the native American succumbed in great numbers, while devising symptomatic remedies. Some tribes were so confused by this "new" disease that they thought it was caused by the beef they had only recently introduced to their diets. As Driver points out, "Their choice of cattle from among the dozens or hundreds of things they had derived from the Whites by that date reflects the persistence of the native notion that animals cause most disease."

Mumps, which is characterized by inflamed parotid glands coupled with headache and fever, was treated in several cases with plants later admitted to the *U.S. Pharmacopoeia* for their sedative and diuretic properties. In this we see the signs of sagacious intuitive medicine. The modern treatment for mumps usually consists of a liquid diet to promote urination (a diuretic encourages this, e.g., red cedar below) and bed rest.

ᴈ RED CEDAR (FIG.73)

The fruit and leaves of red cedar were boiled and the resulting tea taken for coughs, colds, and Asian flu by several Indian tribes, but the Natchez used an unnamed part of this juniper specifically for treating mumps. This is another example of an intelligent, intuitive application because the fresh young twigs of juniper were officially recognized for their diuretic properties and entered in the *U.S. Pharmacopoeia* from 1820 to 1894.

A volatile oil from cedar wood has been used for abortion, and in some cases has caused vomiting convulsions, coma, and death. Red cedar wood oil, which is composed of cedar camphor, or cedrol, is used as a moth repellent and as an insecticide in sprays and dusts. It has also been employed as a scent in the manufacture of soap. Cedar needles have been burned as incense during

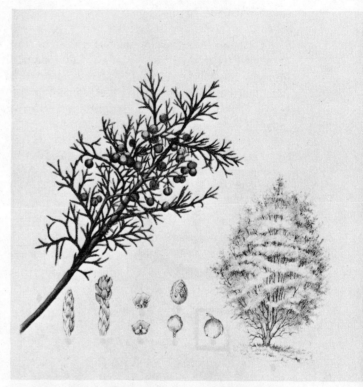

(FIG. 73) RED CEDAR: *A tea made of the fruit and leaves was taken for coughs, colds, and influenza by several tribes, while the Natchez used the plant to treat mumps.*

the peyote meeting among the Kiowa, a Plains tribe.

This evergreen tree attains a height of twenty-five to forty feet in the northern latitudes, while in the south a height of one hundred feet is not uncommon. When young, this species takes on a conical appearance, but the branches spread with age giving a cylindrical outline. The light blue cones are berrylike, about three inches in diameter, and are borne on straight branchlets which are shorter than their own length.

ᴈ HIGHBUSH CRANBERRY

The Malecite Indians ranged geographically from the valley of the St. John River in New

Brunswick into the northeastern part of Maine. Though their origin is thought to be somewhere in the Southwest, their tribal name is derived from the Micmac term, which means "broken talkers." This tribe and the Penobscots of Maine treated mumps by drinking an infusion of an unnamed part of the highbush cranberry. Since it is the bark which most clearly holds the medicinal properties, it is safe to assume that these people discovered this remedy through their own methods.

Cranberry bark was widely used in the United States for its sedative and antispasmodic properties from 1894 through 1916 when it was listed in the *U.S. Pharmacopoeia*. In recognizance of its properties, it was also popularly known as cramp bark. Around 1909, the bark brought a wholesale price of only two to four and one-half cents a pound. An early writer of this century stated that the Indians employed this plant for its diuretic properties, which is interesting because the excretion of liquids is desirable during the course of mumps.

The plant is indigenous to southern Canada and the northern United States. The commerical supplies are gathered from plants growing wild in Maine, Michigan, and Minnesota.

The name of this species, *Opulus*, means "power" or "wealth" and refers to the abundance of foliage of this shrub. The tree grows between eight and ten feet high and has broad, oval leaves of three lobes. The lower leaf surface shows moderately hairy veins while the upper surface is usually smooth. The white flower heads appear in June or July and measure from three to four inches across. The sour red fruits contain a "pit" and resemble the true cranberry in taste and appearance. The bark is still employed for its medicinal properties.

ᴇᴢ SWEET EVERLASTING (FIG.74)

The only tribe to have passed on a use for the sweet everlasting is the Creek. To relieve the swollen glands associated with mumps, they boiled a large quantity of the leaves in water, added lard, dipped cloths in the liquid, and then tied them around the area of swelling.

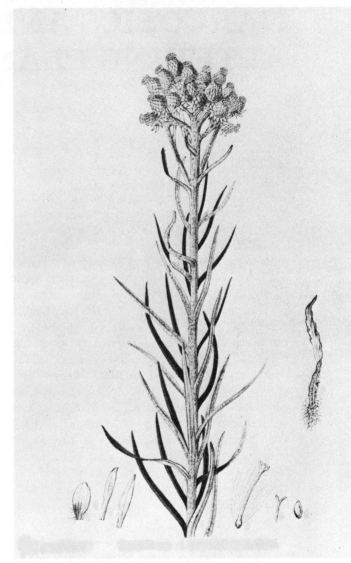

(FIG. 74) SWEET EVERLASTING: *To relieve the swollen glands associated with mumps, the Creeks boiled a large quantity of these leaves in water, added lard, dipped cloths into the liquid, and then tied them around the area of swelling.*

Sweet everlasting grows abundantly in dry meadows alongside roads through a broad geographical sweep—from Newfoundland to Alaska, south to West Virginia and west through California. It is between one and three feet in height and bears pale yellow "flowers" from August to October.

NARCOTICS AND MIND-ALTERING PLANTS

MESCAL BEAN

The mescal bean played a minor role in daily Indian life but was eaten by about a dozen tribes in the United States and Mexico to induce visions during initiation rites. Many Plains Indians used them as the basis for the Red Bean Dance. Today, the Comanche and Kiowa tribes wear the seeds in necklace form as part of the peyote ceremony.

The mescal bean, a member of the bean family, is not at all related to the heads of the peyote cactus which are sometimes referred to as mescal buttons. The seeds of this plant contain a highly poisonous alkaloid called cytisine, which is also known as sophorine. This crystalline alkaloid, which is pharmacologically related to nicotine, acts violently in the human system. Professor Richard Evan Schultes, foremost authority on the subject of hallucinogenic drugs, points out that the mescal bean was dropped as a native narcotic "with the sweeping arrival of peyote which was so much safer and so much more spectacularly hallucinogenic."

BLACK DRINK PLANT

An infusion of the leaves of the small tree black drink plant was used ceremonially by several Indian groups in the southeastern United States. The leaves were first toasted over a fire in a clay vessel and then boiled for several hours after which the thick black liquid was drunk. Ingestion was followed by immediate vomiting, this rite of purification preceding a hunt or war expedition. The Creeks, however, imbibed the black drink during important councils and tribal ceremonies, especially during their yearly harvest ceremony.

The Cultachiches, who inhabited the region west of the mouth of the Mississippi River, excluded women from their ceremony. The following scene, related by an early Spanish explorer in 1564, appears in W. E. Safford's paper in the *Annual Report of the Smithsonian Institution for 1916*:

[The boiling leaves were kept covered] and if by chance it should be uncovered, and a woman should come by in the meantime, they would drink none of it but fling it all away. Likewise while it was cooling and being poured out to drink, no woman was allowed to stir or make a motion, or they would pour it all out on the ground and spew up any which they might have drunk, while she would be severely beaten. All this time they would continue bawling out: "Who will drink?" whereupon the women, on hearing this call, became motionless, and were they sitting or standing, even on tip-toe, or with one leg raised and the other down, they dared not change their position until the men had cooled the liquor and made it ready to drink. The reason they gave for this is quite as foolish and unreasonable as the custom itself; for they said that if the women did not stand still on hearing the call some evil would be imparted to the liquor which they believed would make them die.

It is not difficult to imagine why many of the early white settlers of Florida, Georgia, and the Carolinas adopted this drink. One possibility lies in the fact that the Florida Indians allowed only their bravest warriors the right to drink it. Perhaps some of the early whites attempted to prove their strength to the Indians by partaking of this liquid, later taking to drinking it on a regular basis.

PEYOTE

The peyote plant belongs to the cactus family but is unique botanically in that it lacks spines. The peyote "button" consists of the heads of this small species which are sliced off and dried prior to being eaten or infused in water and then drunk. This plant is used by members of more than thirty Indian tribes. It has replaced almost all plants which were formerly used therapeutically and is considered by many users as a universal panacea. Professor Schultes has summarized various aspects of the peyote cult and traces its introduction to the United States to the Comanche and Kiowa raiding expeditions to Mexico. Professor Schultes summarized the peyote story as follows:

> Another of the sacred plants closely tied in with religious practices which the conquerors of Mexico encountered was the now famous *peyote* cactus, *Lophophora Williamsii*. The spineless heads of this small grey-green cactus with a long carrot-like root are sliced off and dried to form the so-called *mescal buttons*. These buttons contain eight anhalonium alkaloids of the isoquinoline series, all of which have been synthesized. The intoxication induced by eating mescal buttons is one of the most highly complex known and has been too often and expertly described in the literature to detail here. The most spectacular phase of this intoxication is made up of the kaleidoscopic play of richly coloured visual hallucinations, and this phase is attributable to but one of the alkaloids, *mescaline*. It is primarily this extraordinary phase of the narcosis which has convinced Mexican and North American Indians that the plant is a divine messenger enabling the partaker to communicate with the gods without the medium of a priest and has occupied the serious attention of experimental psychologists now for a number of years.

Peyote goes back far in Mexican history. The chronicles of the Conquistadores are full of fanatic and vituperative condemnation of the peyote as a diabolic root. Missionaries combatted its use in native religions as a sacred element and compared the eating of the cactus with cannibalism.

Peyote survived, however, as a divine therapeutic agent and religious hallucinogen in northern Mexico, where the explorer Lumholtz in 1892 discovered its use in ceremonial dances amongst the Huichols and Tarahumares and sent back to Harvard University material upon which a definitive botanical determination was made.

During the last half of the past century, Indian tribes from the United States brought back knowledge of the peyote from their raids into northern Mexico. After 1880, peyote was accepted with great speed amongst many tribes in the United States as the central sacrament in a religious cult which incorporated both Christian and aboriginal

elements. By 1922, the adherents to the peyote cult numbered 13,300 and, for protection against fierce persecution from missionary and governmental circles, it was legally incorporated into the Native American Church. There are now many more tribes and members practicing the cult, which has spread as far north as Saskatchewan.

It may be interesting to include the structural formula of the active principle of this cactus, mescaline.

$$H_3CO \quad CH_2-CH_2-NH_2$$
$$H_3CO \quad OCH_3$$

MESCALINE, the active principle
of the peyote buttons.

⤚§ JIMSON WEED (FIG.75)

Varieties of this genus were taken for their narcotic effect by tribes in California and the southwestern United States, Mexico, and Central and South America. In general, the leaves, stems, and roots were gathered, pounded, and allowed to soak in water for several hours, after which the solution was strained and drunk. Its uses varied between tribes but commonly attracted the interest of users for purposes of divination.

Harold E. Driver, a lifetime student of the ways of the Indians of North America, outlines some of the uses of this plant:

> In California the drug was usually taken at the age of puberty or later by a group of young people under the supervision of elders . . . Where definite male puberty initiations existed, the drinking of *Datura* was a part of these rites . . . A considerable number of California tribes used it as an anesthetic for setting broken bones or otherwise treating the injured. Medicine men also took the drug in order to "see sickness." . . . In the Oasis it was most often taken . . . to bring success on a deer hunt, to alleviate vomiting and dizziness, to induce the drinker to utter prophecies, or simply for the pleasure derived from the accompanying dreams and visions. At Zuñi, *Datura* was believed to be one of the medicines derived from the gods, and its use was limited to rain priests

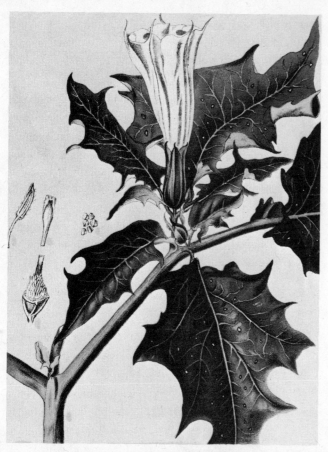

(FIG. 75) JIMSON WEED: *A narcotic tea was taken by tribes in California and the southwestern United States. The leaves contain hyoscyamine and atropine and have been used in American medicine as a sedative and to relieve asthmatic complaints.*

and directors of the Little Fire and Cimex fraternities . . . If a man had been robbed and wished to discover the thief, the priests gave him a dose of *Datura*. Here also it was used as an anesthetic to set fractured bones or perform surgery on a patient. (Driver, *Indians of North America*, pp. 103–104)

The Mohaves and Paiutes employed the plant for similar purposes, while the Mariposa gave the liquid to the young women of their tribe when the reputed aphrodisiac properties were desired.

The origin of the name jimson weed comes to us from Robert Beverly's early history of the state of Virginia. Some of the soldiers sent to Jamestown in 1676 to put down Bacon's Rebellion gathered the young shoots of jimson weed and cooked them as a vegetable,

the Effect of which was a very pleasant Comedy; for they turn'd natural Fools upon it for Several Days: One would blow up a Feather in the Air; another would dart Straws at it with much Fury;

and another stark naked was sitting up in a Corner, like a Monkey, grinning and making Mows at them; a Fourth would fondly kiss, and paw his Companions, and snear in their Faces, with a Countenance more antick, than any in a *Dutch* Droll. In this frantick Condition they were confined, lest they should in their Folly destroy themselves; though it was observed, that all their Actions were full of Innocence and good Nature. Indeed, they were not very cleanly; for they would have wallow'd in their own Excrements, if they had not been prevented. A Thousand such simple Tricks they play'd, and after Eleven Days, return'd themselves again, not remembering any thing that had pass'd. (Beverly, *History of Virginia*, p. 121)

But this was not the first time a group of soldiers had ingested jimson weed. In 37 and 38 B.C., during a retreat, Anthony's legion consumed the plant with equally comic results.

The medical history of this drug plant is described by Dr. Millspaugh, who concluded by suggesting that it was a valuable treatment for rabies!

From the symptoms caused by this drug, its homoeopathic adaptability to hydrophobia will be at once evident. There is no drug so far proven that deserves as thorough and careful a trial in this dread disease as stramonium. The following from a letter written by the Catholic Bishop of Singapore to the *Straits Times*, has just come to my notice. This Bishop says he thinks it is his duty to publish the remedies used in the missions in Tonquin for the cure of hydrophobia. These, he says, consist, first, in giving as much star-aniseed as may be contained on a cent piece; and, secondly, in making the patient take some water in which a handful of the leaves of stramony, or thorn-apple, or pear-apple, is infused. These will cause an access of the convulsions or delirium, during which the patient must be tied; but on its abatement he will be cured. If the remedy act too violently, either by too much being administered, or on account of there being no virus of real hydrophobia, the consequences may be ameliorated by making the patient drink an infusion of licorice root, a most precious antidote against poisoning by stramony. In 1869, the Bishop relates, a very honorable member of the clergy of Paris was bitten by a pet dog, which died thirty hours afterwards with the most characterized convulsions of rabies. The following day he felt the first symptoms of the dreadful disease, and these augmented in intensity every day. The priest, however, applied at once all sorts of known remedies, ancient and modern, and even employed a very small dose of stramony. Each time he used the latter the progress of the disease ceased for some hours, even days, and then continued its ravages with greater intensity than before. When the fatal issue was at hand, just at the crisis of the disease, when the paroxysms had attained the greatest violence, the patient, with almost super-human energy, began chewing a pinch of dried stramony leaves, swallowing the juice. The effect was not long in making itself felt. In half an hour the disease had attained its height, the patient being delirious during the convulsions; but on the following day he was perfectly cured. "The same remedy," concludes the Bishop, "is used in India, and is always successful." (Millspaugh, *Medicinal Plants*, 1887, pp. 127–5 to 127–6)

From the same author we learn the origin of the word *thug*, "a society of stealthy fanatic murderers of India" who employed varieties of jimson weed to "render their intended victims unconscious."

At that time in America, jimson weed leaves were smoked to alleviate asthmatic attacks, and as an ointment they were applied to burns and scalds. At the beginning of this century the leaves were known for their narcotic, diuretic, antispasmodic, and pain-relieving properties.

The main constituents of stramonium leaves are similar to belladonna leaves, namely, hyoscyamine and atropine. There are also traces of scopolamine, a potent cholinergic-blocking hallucinogen that has been used in medicine to calm excited schizoid patients and in childbirth to induce sleep with amnesia. Surprisingly, this powerful drug is available on a nonprescription basis in a sleeping compound called Sominex. How is it that so much is said about marijuana, a relatively mild drug—one that carries with it all the threats of illegality—when scopolamine, a much stronger psychotomimetic, is available over the counter?

Hyoscyamine and atropine act to inhibit the parasympathetic nervous system, which characteristically results in drying of the mucous membranes of the mouth, bronchial tree, and stomach, and relaxation of smooth muscle of the alimentary and bronchial tracts. The *Dispensatory of the United States* for 1942 states that the leaves are used in the treatment of asthma and "the beneficial effect is doubtless due to the presence of atropine which paralyzes the endings of the pulmonary branch of the vagus, thus relieving the bronchial spasm. . . ."

The leaves and flowering tops of jimson weed were official in the *U.S. Pharmacopoeia* from 1820 to 1950 and in the *National Formulary* from 1950 to 1965. They were primarily used for asthmatic complaints.

Before leaving this narcotic species, I would like once again to turn to an observer of the past in an attempt to encourage our present pharmacologists and psychologists to search the plant world for a drug capable of restoring sanity to a mad person.

Baron Störck, of Vienna, introduced jimson weed to the medical profession in 1762. He used the drug in epilepsy and insanity and questioned:

> If Stramonium produces symptoms of madness in a healthy person, would it not be desirable to make experiments in order to discover whether this plant . . . would not restore to a healthy state those who are suffering from alienation of mind?

Jimson weed is thought to be indigenous to Europe, possibly to the borders of the Caspian Sea, but another school of botanists believes the plant may be indigenous to several countries. It grows as an uncultivated weed in South America, southern Russia, and Asia, while in the United States it grows near waste heaps where the soil is rich and loose. The Indians originally named it the white man's plant, referring to its habitat—garbage dumps.

This member of the nightshade family has stout, yellowish green stems about two to five feet high and large leaves, from three to eight inches long, that are wavy-toothed, dark green above and lighter green on the lower surface. The large, white, trumpet-shaped flowers appear from May to September. These are followed by seed pods which burst open, expressing black poisonous seeds. When used for the constituents, the leaves and tops are collected when the plant is in flower and carefully dried.

It should be remembered that any plant may be "safe" for one person and poisonous, even fatal, to another.

Aside from the above narcotics and the mushrooms found in Mexico which contain psilocybin, there are other lesser-known plants with reputed narcotic effects that were employed in Indian therapeutics or ceremonials.

The Indians of the northwestern United States chewed a fern *Lycopodium selago* for its narcotic-like effects. By chewing the stems of three plants, a mild intoxication was experienced, while chew-

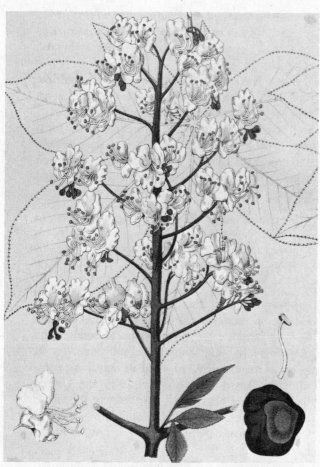

(FIG. 76) HORSE CHESTNUT: *The nuts of this tree were used as a narcotic during the nineteenth century and were considered by some physicians to be equal in effect to opium.*

ing those of eight plants was said to render the individual unconscious.

The Calpella Indians of northern Calfornia considered the root of red larkspur to contain "highly narcotic properties" and referred to the plant as sleeproot.

In concluding this brief summary of narcotic plants, we include a minor narcotic of our grandfather's generation. Dr. Millspaugh describes the nuts of the horse chestnut (FIG. 76) as narcotic and states that "10 grains are equal to 3 grams of opium." Surprisingly, the pulverized nuts were mixed with lard by the Indians and used as a home remedy for hemorrhoids. Some California Indians employed a related species as an agent for suicide, evidence that each culture employs their narcotic drugs in their own way.

NIPPLES (Sore)

BALSAM FIR

The Indians utilized the resins of the spreading balsam fir tree on cuts, wounds, and burns. This bark exudate, which has also been named Canada balsam, was formerly employed in domestic medicine as a cooling application for sore nipples. (The plant is treated in greater detail under "Burns.") The balsam fir, common in the Northeast, is easily recognized by its needles which are dark green above and whitened on the underside. The cones are violet or purplish when young and are smooth and cylindric in shape. About 30 percent of all Christmas trees cut and sold each year are of this species.

MILK PURSLANE (COMMON SPURGE)

The Cherokees prepared an ointment of the milk purslane species (probably by combining the bruised root with animal fat) and rubbed the mixture in for skin sores and sore nipples. Plants of this genus were frequently employed to induce vomiting; however, in strong doses this emetic action was associated with vertigo, dimness of vision, and heat flashes. This species generally irritates mucous membranes and may act as acrid poisons.

This annual herb grows between eight and eighteen inches high, contains a milky juice, and has numerous white or red flowers. Indigenous to North America, it is generally found growing in dry fields, or cultivated grounds, and on hillsides, where it flowers from July to September.

WHITE TRILLIUM (FIG. 77)

The Potawatomi tribe of lower Michigan pounded the root of the attractive white trillium lily and steeped the pulped mass in water, utilizing the liquid as a wash for sore nipples. A wet dressing of the freshly dug root was used on eye inflammations by the Menominees. Early white settlers named this plant birth root or beth root

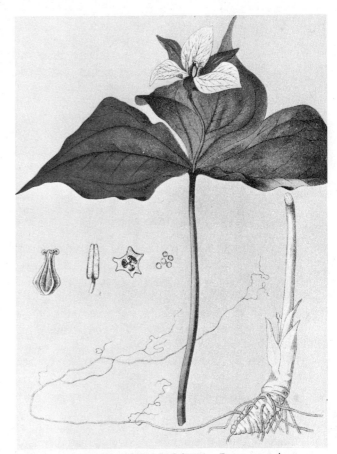

(FIG. 77) WHITE TRILLIUM: *The Potawatomis prepared a wash from the root of this attractive lily to soothe sore nipples in nursing women.*

because it was then popularly held that the Indians employed it to induce labor in childbirth. The Indians of Canada and Missouri employed the roots to cure vaginal discharge, to retard profuse menstruation, and to stop bleeding following parturition. Subsequently, all common species of white trillium became popular in domestic medicine, being employed internally for uterine hemorrhage and externally for their tonic, astringent, and antiseptic properties.

The dried roots and rhizome of *Trillium erectum* were entered in the *National Formulary* from 1916 to 1947, when they were used for various purposes, not one of which is today accepted.

NOSEBLEED

❧ GIANT BIRD'S NEST

The Cheyennes mixed the ground stem and berries of giant bird's nest in boiling water and snuffed the liquid after it was cooled. They named this species nosebleed medicine and also drank the same preparation for bleeding of the lungs. There is no other record ascribing any medicinal use for this plant. (For a detailed description of a related plant, see Indian pipe under "Eye Problems.")

❧ BIRD'S-FOOT FERN

With one exception, there is little reported Indian use of ferns in medicine. Robert M. Lloyd, an expert on ferns of North America, researched this topic and reported that the Minok tribe snuffed an infusion of the steeped fronds of the bird's-foot fern to arrest nosebleeds. His very interesting paper on ferns of California lists the economic and medicinal uses of twenty-two fern species.

❧ PULSATILLA (FIG. 78)

The Thompson Indians of British Columbia named this or a closely related species bleeding nose plant. A bunch of pulsatilla blossoms was held to the nostrils or the leaves were inserted until bleeding subsided. Several varieties were employed by Indian practitioners in treating boils, burns, sore eyes, and wounds.

Pulsatilla was formerly used in the United States by eclectic physicians for treating sterility and infected ovaries. The drug, which is derived from the chopped whole plant, is known to induce vomiting and irritation of the kidneys. In high dosage it acts as a depressant on the central nervous system and heart. The above-named species was official in the *U.S. Pharmacopoeia* from 1882 to 1905 and was utilized for its diuretic, expectorant, and menstrual-inducing qualities.

The genus name, *Anemone*, means "wind" in Greek; this beautiful "wind flower," as it was also

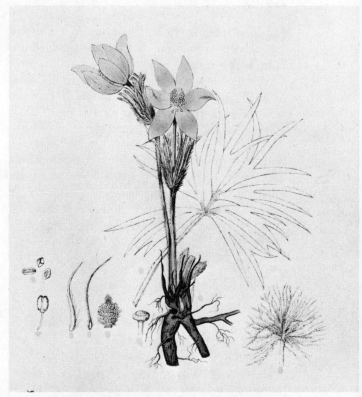

(FIG. 78) PULSATILLA: *The Thompson Indians of British Columbia used this as their "bleeding nose plant." To stop bleeding, a bunch of blossoms was held to the nostrils.*

called, grows from four to ten inches tall and bears a white to purple flower about two inches across. It is frequent on the prairies from Wisconsin north, and west to the Rocky Mountains. It usually flowers around Eastertime, which is the reason it is sometimes referred to as pasque flower. The drug was collected at the time of flowering, and the whole plant chopped and dried.

❧ BUTTON SNAKEROOT (FIG. 79)

Both species of button snakeroot were widely used by the Indians of North America. The Natchez of Mississippi inserted the chewed stem and leaves into their nostrils to stop nosebleed, while other tribes valued an infusion of the pounded root for reducing fevers. The root was used for its diuretic properties by the Meskwaki, while the Creeks utilized a drink of button snakeroot to induce vomiting prior to a hunt or before important ceremonies. For the same emetic purposes, the Koasati Indians drank a decoction of the boiled root.

C. F. Millspaugh, in his classic work, reported that following its use by the Indians, button snakeroot was adopted as a folk remedy and then accepted by physicians for its stimulant, diuretic, and expectorant properties. He also reported that a tea of the boiled root "has been found useful in dropsy, nephritic and calculous disorders; chronic laryngitis and bronchitis; irritation of the urethra, vaginal, uterine, and cystic mucous membranes; gonorrhea, gleet, and leucorrhea; muccoid diarrhea; local inflammations of the mucous membranes; exhaustion from sexual depletion with loss of erectile power, seminal emissions, and orchitis."

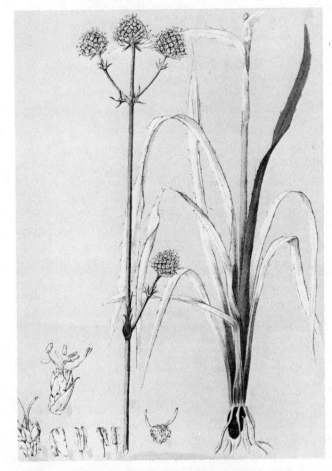

(FIG. 79) BUTTON SNAKEROOT: *To stop nosebleed, the Natchez of Mississippi inserted the chewed stem and leaves into their nostrils.*

PARALYSIS

There is no evidence which suggests that paralysis was common among the native Americans. The life expectancy of aboriginal American Indians has been estimated at thirty-seven years by an anthropologist who analyzed skeletal remains. Since paralysis is common in older people who have suffered from cerebral "strokes," it is unlikely that this affliction caused the Indian much concern and therefore it is equally unlikely that any of the following plant "remedies" for paralysis had any beneficial effect. Nevertheless, these plant medicines are included for historical purposes and to broaden the spectrum of "Indian remedies."

❧ PEARLY EVERLASTING

To treat a victim of paralysis, the Flambeau Ojibwas first crushed and then burned the pearly white blossoms of this species and encouraged the patient to inhale the smoke.

There is no record which indicates wide acceptance for this plant in American medicine; however, the *Dispensatory of the United States* for 1942 states that everlasting:

> is sometimes used in the form of tea in intestinal and pulmonary catarrhs, and, externally, in the way of fomentation, in bruises, but it probably possesses little medicinal virtue. In Europe different species . . . are occasionally employed for similar purposes.

This snow-white, fuzzy plant, has an erect stem which grows between one and three feet in height. It has very narrow leaves that are white and fuzzy on the lower surface. The pearly white blossoms appear between July and September. Pearly everlasting is found throughout southern Canada and the northern United States south to West Virginia.

❧ AMERICAN SENNA

Senna leaves are best known for their laxative effects; this plant is described in detail under that heading. For some reason, the Cherokees treated paralysis by drinking a tea of pounded senna root.

❧ WINTERGREEN

The Montagnais, a people of Labrador and southeastern Canada, drank wintergreen tea to treat paralysis. We know these people by a French name which means "mountaineers," a reference to the geographical structure of their native lands. The Indians referred to themselves, however, as *Ne-e-no-il-no*, which J. R. Swanton translates as meaning "perfect people." They also called themselves "people of the north-northeast," which indicates their awareness of the great tribes of the area now bounded by the United States.

POISON IVY AND POISON OAK

SWEET FERN

To cure the effects of poison ivy the Mohegans steeped the frondlike sweet fern leaves in water and rubbed in the liquid as a cooling wash. The plant has been used in American medicine but for a different purpose—mainly for tonic and astringent purposes and to cure diarrhea.

Sweet fern was so named because of the resemblance of its leaves to the spleenwort fern and for its fragrant odor. It is a shrubby indigenous plant with reddish brown bark and grows from about one to three feet in height. The narrow leaves are fernlike, about three to six inches long, and deeply divided into many lobes. Sweet fern belongs to the bayberry family and is usually found on dry hillsides in Canada and the northeastern United States.

GUM PLANT

Indian tribes of northern California applied the pounded sappy leaves of the gum plant for ivy poisoning and also used the resinous gum to relieve asthma, bronchitis, and whooping cough. In 1863, a Dr. Canfield of Monterey, California, reported that the Indians used gum plant for poison ivy rash. By 1875, the plant was introduced into official American medicine. The dried leaves and flowering tops of various species were official in the *U.S. Pharmacopoeia* from 1882 to 1926 and in the *National Formulary* from 1926 to 1960. The plant is used as a sedative, as an antispasmodic, and in the form of a fluid extract, in the treatment of ivy poisoning. The fluid extract is prepared by placing the freshly gathered leaves and flowers in a small amount of simmering water for about fifteen minutes. This extract is pharmacologically equal to commerical preparations of the gum.

The gum plant is very common in the western and central desert regions of California. In Oregon, the Willamette Valley region is conspicuously covered with gum plant during the summer when the yellow flowers begin to appear. The gum is collected before the flowers have opened, when the white sticky gum envelops the buds and leaves.

The gum plant has a round, smooth stem and grows about eighteen inches in height. The leaves are broad and round at their perimeters and narrow toward their bases. They are leathery, pale green, toothed, and about one inch long. The gum plant has several branches toward the top, each of which terminates in a large, yellow flower.

The leaves and flowering tops are collected just as the flowers are in full bloom, during the summer months. The gum has a balsamic odor and a bitter taste.

SOAPROOT

The Pomo Indians of Mendocino County prepared a lotion of the soapy juice from the roots of soaproot and rubbed it on the rash of poison oak.

MILK VETCH

The Cheyennes ground the leaves and stems of the milk vetch, their "poisonweed medicine," until it was composed of very fine pieces and sprinkled the powder on poison ivy rashes that had become watery. A European relative (A. *exscapus*) was once popularly prescribed in decoction for syphilitic sores. In 1832, William Woodville—an English physician who authored a brilliant five-volume edition on medical botany—wrote about the stemless milk vetch:

> Since the year 1786 this plant has been much celebrated as a remedy in syphilitic complaints . . . By persevering a few weeks in the use of this decoction . . . without mercury, the various symptoms of the most inveterate syphilis, as nodes, exostoses, tophi, scabies, venereal blotches, buboes, ulcers, etc. have been effectually cured.

JEWELWEED (TOUCH-ME-NOT)

The Potawatomi Indians applied the juice from the leaves of this touch-me-not to relieve the itch caused by ivy poisoning. To cure rashes and eczema, the Omahas applied the crushed leaves and stem. The Blackfoot Indians treated rashes and eczema by applying the mashed stems and leaves of a related species of touch-me-not, *I. capensis*.

Jewelweed grows to a height of five or six feet and bears yellowish flowers which hang by slender stalks. They have capsules which burst and curl up on the slightest touch. This succulent species is indigenous to low, moist, shaded areas and is found from Newfoundland to Alaska and south to Florida.

⁊ WORMWOOD

The Yokia Indians of Mendocino County used unnamed parts of the wormwood plant specifically for treating the effects of poison oak.

To treat the effects of poison ivy rash the Omahas prepared the fruits and leaves of smooth upland sumac and applied the mash in the form of a wet dressing. As a last-named species used for this rash, we once again come to the wild lettuce. The Menominees rubbed in the milky juice from a freshly picked plant to cure the cutaneous eruptions of ivy poisoning.

RATTLESNAKE BITE

The many remedies used for bites of snakes, in general, are treated under "Snakebite." Under the present heading are listed those plants used by some Indian tribes specifically against the effects of the bite of a rattlesnake. Since, with the exception of white ash, these plants were not borrowed by the early settlers, there is little information about them in the literature. Consequently, the plants are listed without reference to later applications, assays, etc.

⋑ WHITE ASH (FIG. 80)

The white ash enjoyed some popularity in early domestic medicine as an Indian remedy for the bite of the rattlesnake. Dr. Millspaugh, quoting Dr. Porcher, who quoted "some unmentioned author" wrote in 1887:

> The leaves of this plant are said to be so highly offensive to the rattlesnake, that that formidable reptile is never found on land where it grows; and it is the practice of hunters and others, having occasion to traverse the woods in the summer months, to stuff their boots or shoes with WHITE ASH leaves, as a preventative of the bite of the rattlesnake.

Dr. Millspaugh further states that the early settlers of Orange County, New York, carried the leaves for the same purpose. He cautions us, however, against believing "in this prophylactic."

Reports of this sort appeared as early as 1794. As we learn from Virgil J. Vogel's work, Loskiel, the missionary, wrote: "A decoction of the buds or bark of the *white ash* (*fraxinus Carolina*) taken inwardly is said to be a certain remedy against the effects of this poison."

Aside from the facts that white ash bark was used in medicine for its tonic and astringent properties and that it was official in the *National Formulary* from 1916 to 1926, the main attraction of this species has been as an important source of lumber. It is interesting to imagine how an early American Indian, who believed in the rattlesnake-

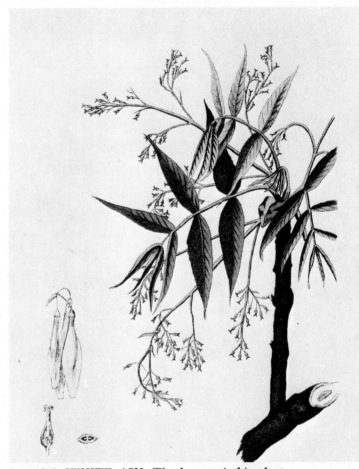

(FIG. 80) WHITE ASH: *The leaves of this plant were once very popular in the United States as rattlesnake deterrents. Hunters, who are said to have learned about this plant from the Indians, once stuffed their boots with white ash leaves.*

repelling qualities of this tree, would react if he came upon a mill that was turning out tool handles and furniture from an otherwise divine medicinal species.

⋑ PTILORIA

The Zuñi of New Mexico first sucked out the toxin and then applied a powder of the ground plant on the bite. This treatment was

111

repeated on four consecutive mornings. The patient was instructed to eat sparingly and drink only small quantities of water into which a bit of the same root powder was dissolved. This treatment was employed specifically for the bites of the rattlesnake, the Zuñi having other remedies for the bites of other venomous snakes.

The Navajos applied a wet dressing of the pounded leaves of beardtongue to rattlesnake bite, and their lore considers this treatment to be "an absolute antidote."

When the Thompson Indians of British Columbia ventured into territories which were host to rattlers, the spurge common to that region of Canada became an item of special value for their medicine bags. If bitten, the Thompson crushed the stem and applied the milky juice directly on the wound.

RESPIRATORY PROBLEMS

❧ ELECAMPANE (FIG. 81)

The only record of Indian employment of the strikingly beautiful herb elecampane appears in a book of remedies written in 1870 by a folk-healer, John Goodale Briante, who claimed to have lived for several years with the Potawatomis and the "St. Francis Tribe of Indians, at Green Bay." One authority (Vogel) believes that Mr. Briante's "remedy" was not of Indian origin because the Indians seldom combined more than three plants in any mixture and this particular syrup was made by combining nine herbs, one of which was elecampane. Nevertheless, elecampane is discussed here because it had been used for a long while in European medicine, later becoming an official medicine in the United States, for respiratory ailments.

Hippocrates, termed by some the father of medicine, stated that elecampane was a stimulant to the uterus, kidneys, stomach, and brain. This may also be the *Helenium foliis verbasci* of Dioscorides, and the *Inula* of Pliny. It was once widely used in English medicine as a diuretic and as an agent to induce profuse sweating, but later fell into disuse. Elecampane was one of the substances used in France in the preparation of absinthe, a liqueur which is described in the section on "Bronchitis."

Clinical experiments indicate that an extract of this plant is a powerful antiseptic and bactericide that is particularly effective against the organism which causes tuberculosis. The dried root, official in the *U.S. Pharmacopoeia*, was used in "affections of the respiratory organs," in skin diseases, and in digestive and liver disorders. A textbook on plant drugs that was published in 1936 states that elecampane is a stimulant that was used to promote the expulsion of phlegm (expectorant), to induce sweating (diaphoretic), and to promote the excretion of urine (diuretic).

Although elecampane was originally introduced from Europe as a cultivated plant, it has naturalized itself in the eastern United States west to Missouri and Minnesota and is found along roadsides and in damp pastures and fields. It resembles

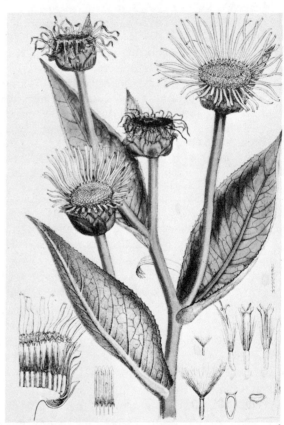

(FIG. 81) ELECAMPANE: *Clinical experiments indicate that an extract of this plant is a powerful antiseptic and bactericide that is particularly effective against the organism which causes tuberculosis.*

the sunflower but grows only from three to six feet in height. The yellow flower appears as illustrated and blossoms between July and September. The roots were collected for medicinal purposes in the fall of the second year of the plant's growth, but not later. This assured the drug dealer of a smooth, solid root that brought him a premium price on the wholesale market.

❧ YERBA SANTA

"No plant is more highly valued as a medicine by all the tribes of Mendocino County." So wrote V. K. Chestnut, in his valuable paper on plant usage by the Indians of that county in California. He continues:

It is found in every household either in the dry state or in whisky extract. It was early adopted by the Spanish missionaries, . . . being of special value in chronic subacute inflammation of the bronchial tubes, and as a means of disguising the taste of quinine. . . . The Indians have various methods of using the plant, and apply it generally in their practice of medicine. The leaf is the only part used. As a cure for colds and for asthma it is considered a specific by the native whites and Indians. It was extensively and very successfully used in Round Valley in the winter of 1897–98 as a cure for grippe, that disease having been especially prevalent at that time. It is generally valued as a blood purifier, a cure for rheumatism, consumption, and catarrh. . . . For the first two diseases the tea is taken freely as a drink for several days.

Yerba santa was introduced to the medical profession in 1875 by an eclectic physician, Dr. J. H. Bundy. It was soon after researched by Parke-Davis & Co., and was adopted as an official drug in the *U.S. Pharmacopoeia* in 1894 where it remained until 1905. It was reentered in 1916 and again dropped in 1947. Since 1947, yerba santa has been recognized and described in the *National Formulary* where it is described as a useful expectorant. The leaves contain a bitter resin, a small amount of volatile oil, and tannic acid.

This evergreen shrub grows on dry hillsides throughout Mendocino County. The smooth stem grows to a height of three to four feet and exudes a gummy substance. The leaves are dark green, oblong or oval in shape, leathery with toothed margins, and grow from three to four inches in length. The white to pale blue flowers appear at the top of the plant in clusters. Other common names for this species include mountain balm, wild balsam, gum leaves, and tar weed.

ST.-JOHN'S-WORT (FIG. 82)

The Menominee tribe combined the rapidly spreading perennial St.-John's-wort with black raspberry root in hot water and drank the resulting tea as a treatment for tuberculosis.

St.-John's-wort was introduced to the United States from Europe, where it had been used in

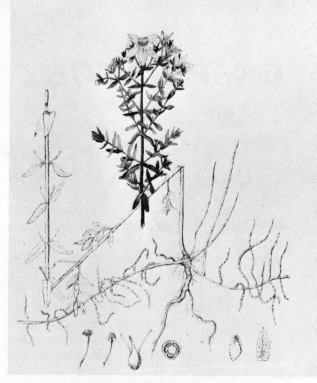

(FIG. 82) *ST.-JOHN'S-WORT: The Menominee tribe combined this perennial weed with black raspberry root in hot water and drank the tea as a treatment for tuberculosis.*

medicine since ancient times. Galen and Dioscorides recommended it as a diuretic, as an emmenagogue, and for killing internal worms. Gerarde, a famous herbalist, says, "St. John's Wort, with his flowers and seed boyled and drunken, provoketh urine, and is right good against stone in the bladder. . . ." The plant received its name from superstitious European peasants who assigned it magical powers and gathered it on St. John's Day for special cures. In the last century it was widely employed as an application to wounds where the nerves were exposed. Millspaugh said, "It is to the nervous system what *Arnica* is to the muscular."

Dr. Eric Stone, the physician who authored an authoritative book on American Indian medicine, states that the Indian practitioner distinguished only the common cold from other respiratory diseases. Bronchitis, pleurisy, and lung affections were all treated with the same medicine, mainly the pleurisy root, yerba santa, mesquite, the sunflower and red cedar. Dr. Stone continues, "One exception was the Sac and Fox group which recognized pleurisy as such and were so far ahead of their time that as early as 1750 they treated pleurisy with effusion by incision and drainage."

RHEUMATISM

Because they were constantly exposed to the weather, the Indians suffered from rheumatism to a considerable extent. Botanical remedies were frequently employed, and some of them will be described, but sweat baths were particularly favored. That of the Yokias of California as described by V. K. Chestnut is included as an interesting example.

These people . . . have a novel way of using the small twigs and leaves for the cure of rheumatism and for bodily bruises. A fire is built over some rocks and allowed to burn down. The pine twigs are then thrown upon the warm ashes and the patient, wrapped well in blankets, lies down upon them. Water is occasionally sprinkled on the rocks beneath, so that steam together with the volatile oil from the leaves is constantly given off. After inhaling this and sweating most profusely for eight or ten hours, the patient is said to be invariably able to move without pain.

The species of pine mentioned in the above account of the Yokia sweat bath is the well-known digger pine. The same tribe sometimes employed the leaves of Douglas fir or wormwood in this cure for rheumatism.

Some of the plants used as remedies for this disorder include the following.

POKEWEED (FIG. 83)

The American Indians utilized the smooth perennial pokeweed as an emetic; however, at least one tribe, the Pamunkey Indians of Virginia, drank a tea of the boiled berries to cure rheumatism. It was borrowed from the Indians and adopted in domestic medicine where the root was applied for various skin diseases.

The dried root of poke was official in the *U.S. Pharmacopoeia* from 1820 to 1916; it was used to relieve pain and to allay inflammation. It has also been employed in chronic rheumatism. Pokeweed is presently being evaluated for its snail-killing properties. A related species, which is found in

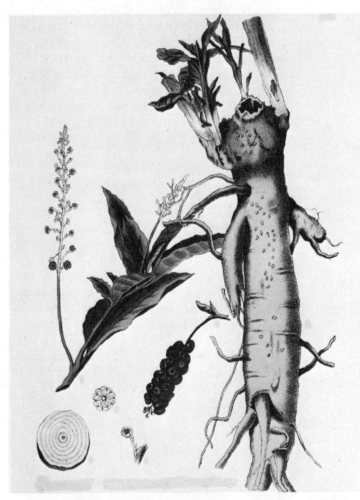

(FIG. 83) POKEWEED: *The Pamunkey Indians of Virginia drank a tea made by boiling the berries to cure rheumatism.*

Africa, has shown molluscicidal properties and the American pokeweed, it is hoped, will be useful in the control of fresh-water snails.

According to the *Dispensatory of the United States*, the dried root has been used in domestic American medicine in the treatment of skin parasites and rheumatism. The fruit juice has been used to treat hemorrhoids, cancer, and tremors.

Appalachian folk practitioners have employed pokeweed berry wine to treat rheumatism. The

Pennsylvania Dutch used the plant for its laxative properties.

This is a common, native weed that is found in moist soil in the eastern and central United States. The long-stalked clusters of white flowers begin to appear in July, and its beautiful bunches of purple berries appear in the fall.

The stems and sprouts of young plants are sometimes boiled in two changes of water and eaten as cooked greens, like asparagus. Poisoning has resulted when inexperienced "naturalists" have eaten pokeweed without proper boiling. The berries have been used in pies, but in the uncooked state should be considered unsafe for children.

✑ BLOODROOT (PUCCOON) (FIG.84)

Bloodroot was a favorite rheumatism remedy among the Indians of the Mississippi region. In Virginia, the Rappahannocks drank a tea of the root for rheumatism, while other tribes used it to induce vomiting.

The bloodroot became popular in domestic American medicine as a stimulating expectorant and was official in the U.S. Pharmacopoeia from 1820 to 1926.

This plant, which belongs to the same family as the opium poppy, contains alkaloids of the protopine series. All these alkaloids are found in other members of the poppy family.

Bloodroot grows in rich open woodlands east of the Mississippi. The waxy white blossoms are among the first of the spring flowers to appear. The generic name, *Sanguinaria*, means "bloody," which refers to the blood-red juice contained in the stem and root.

When used for medicine the rhizome was collected in the fall after the leaves had withered. It was stored in a dry place because moisture encourages deterioration.

The Indians used the red juice to dye their faces and implements, but we are cautioned

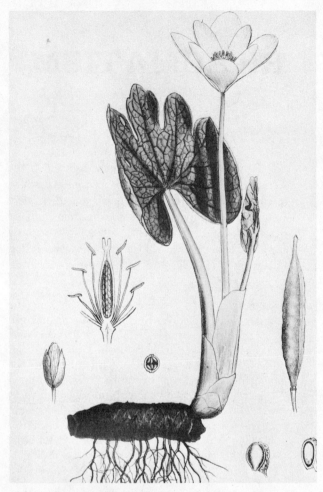

(FIG. 84) BLOODROOT: *This member of the poppy family was a favorite rheumatism remedy among the Indians of the Mississippi region.*

against attempting to eat the rootstock, whether cooked or not. In large quantities it is said to produce poisoning.

Some other plants taken for rheumatism include the plantain, the green leaves of which were applied on the chest as a poultice by the Shoshoni; black cohosh, a decoction of which was taken by the Winnebagos and the Dakotas; and the California polypody fern. The Indians of Mendocino County rubbed the juice from the bruised rhizome of this fern on the regions of rheumatic pain.

RINGWORM

✑ RED BIRCH

The Catawba Indians prepared a salve of red birch by boiling the buds of this tree until they were thick and pasty and then adding sulphur. This salve was applied externally to skin sores and ringworm.

An oil derived from a related species of birch is used as a medicine to kill parasites and as an antiseptic lotion for skin diseases.

✑ POISON IVY (FIG.85)

To cure ringworm the Indians of southern California applied a mash of poison ivy leaves. Some tribes used this plant to promote the suppuration of swellings.

Although this plant causes a well-known skin irritation, it was first used as a medicine in Europe precisely for an opposite effect. A man who accidentally came in contact with the leaves and cured himself of a herpes infection on his wrist, one that he had lived with for six years, reported his marvel to a physician, Du Fresnoy. The plant was soon adopted in general practice to treat difficult herpes infections!

✑ MULBERRY (FIG.86)

The Rappahannocks of Virginia applied the milky latex of the axis of the leaves of red mulberry to the scalp to cure ringworm. In Europe the root bark was boiled in water and the strained decoction taken to kill tapeworms. All the species

(FIG. 86) MULBERRY: *The Rappahannocks of Virginia applied the milky latex of the leaves of red mulberry to the scalp to cure ringworm.*

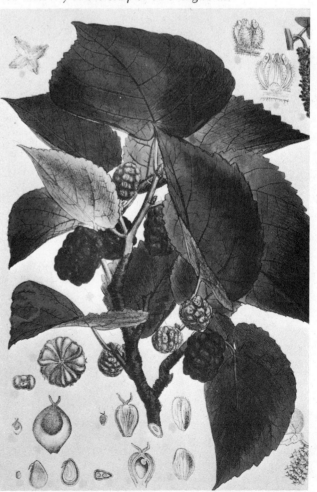

(FIG. 85) POISON IVY: *To cure ringworm the Indians of southern California applied a mash of poison ivy leaves.*

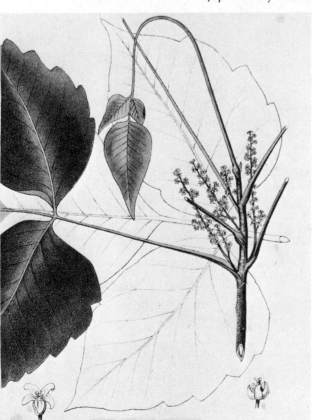

of mulberry have been used for their laxative properties.

Aside from bloodroot, which was used by the Iroquois to treat ringworm, the only other plant listed as a specific Indian botanical for this infection is the tall milkweed. The milky latex was rubbed on by the Rappahannocks of Virginia.

Other plants that were used to cure ringworm will be found in "Skin Problems."

SCURVY

One of the most famous of all Indian "cures" occurred in 1535 when the French explorer Jacques Cartier had lost twenty-five of his men to scurvy and was then icebound in the St. Lawrence River, near the site of the future city of Montreal. Cartier contacted a group of Indians who were walking on the ice near his ship and shrewdly asked for their aid in treating this disease without letting them know the poor health of his remaining crew members. There is still some doubt as to exactly which tree was used to cure his men, for in his journals it is written, "the tree is in their language called Ameda or Hanneda, this is thought to be the Sassafras tree." Several writers believe that an early translator of Cartier's account probably inserted the name of the tree on his own.

Some authorities on Indian medicine believe that the tree was either white pine or hemlock.

Dr. Millspaugh lists the antiscorbutic tree as black spruce (FIG. 87) and definitely states in his work on medicinal plants that "the discoverers of Canada were cured of the scurvy by it, since which it has become in common use in Canada, the Northern States, and even in Europe."

Cartier describes the preparation of this remedy in a section entitled, "How by the grace of God we had notice of a certaine tree, whereby we all recovered our health: and the manner how to use it." An Indian chief, Domagaia,

> sent two women to fetch some of it, which brought ten or twelve branches of it, and therewithall shewed the way how to use it, and that is thus, to take the barke and leaves of the sayd tree, and boile them togither, then to drinke of the sayd decoction every other day, and to put the dregs of it upon his legs that is sicke:

The remedy worked so well on the first few men who tried it that soon fighting broke out

> about who should be first to take it, that they were ready to kill one another, so that a tree as big as any Oake in France was spoiled and lopped bare, and . . . it wrought so wel, that if all the phisicians of Mountpelier and Lovaine had bene

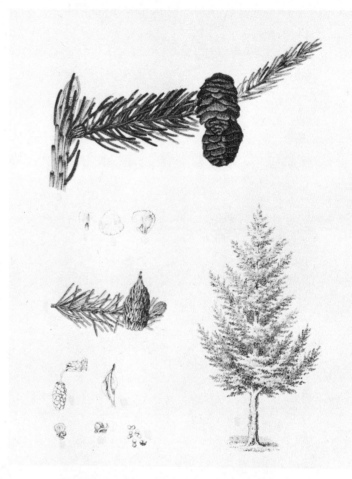

(FIG. 87) *BLACK SPRUCE: Cartier's men were saved from scurvy when they drank a tea made from the leaves of this common conifer.*

> there with all the drugs of Alexandria, they would not have done so much in one yere, as that tree did in six days. . . .

Sprucebeer is still used in the northern regions, and the original Indian formula still holds. The twigs and cones of spruces are boiled in maple syrup and taken hot as a refreshing year-round drink. This drink was also used by Captain Cook on one of his voyages to prevent scurvy and also reappears in American folk medicine as a preventative for this vitamin deficiency.

Other plants which have been used to prevent or cure scurvy include the wild garlic of which the fresh bulbs and green shoots were eaten uncooked; the buds of balsam poplar; the berries of American mountain ash; persimmon leaves, which are said to be high in vitamin C; the bearberry; the highbush cranberry; and all the pine trees. The bright green, young needles were steeped in boiling water for an aromatic tea that is still enjoyed today by people of the outdoors.

It should be remembered that the early American Indians did not suffer from this vitamin C deficiency because they knew how to prevent its occurrence. For the Indians, the above-listed "remedies" were of a preventative nature.

SEDATIVES

WILD BLACK CHERRY

The Indian uses of the popular medicinal plant wild black cherry have already been enumerated under the categories of "Childbirth," "Coughs," "Diarrhea," and "Hemorrhoids." The Meskwaki tribe made a sedative tea of the root bark, and this drink has long been popular in domestic American medicine.

All parts of this plant yield hydrocyanic acid when steeped in water. The medicinal properties of wild cherry are destroyed by boiling; thus the plant is allowed to soak only in warm water.

The bark has been in the U.S. *Pharmacopoeia* since 1820 and has been used as a sedative and in cough medicines.

The wild cherry tree sometimes grows taller than ninety feet and attains a trunk diameter of four feet. The straight trunk is covered with a rough, black bark, and the leaves are bright green above and hairy on the lower surface. Numerous small, white, five-petaled flowers appear on the ends of leafy branches during summer, and the cherries ripen in late August or early September. When used in medicines, the bark is collected in autumn when it contains the greatest concentration of precursors to hydrocyanic acid. Alice Henkel, an early expert on medicinal plants, cautioned against storing the bark for longer than one year, stating that it deteriorates with time. She added that young, thin bark was preferred and that bark from small or old branches was discarded.

PASSIONFLOWER

The Houma Indians added the pulverized root of the indigenous passionflower herb to their water, believing that it acted as a systemic tonic. Although this plant was used to some extent by Indians of South America, it did not receive very much attention in North American medical circles until the latter part of the nineteenth century when the flowering and fruiting tops were used to relieve insomnia and to soothe nerves.

Little is known about the pharmacology of this plant; however, it is an ingredient in several commercial drug preparations.

The passionflower is named for its large flowers which supposedly represented the passion of Jesus to the early Spanish explorers of this continent. The plants, found throughout the southern United States, produce their flowers from May to July. The drug is collected for medicines after some of the yellowish fruits, which are about the size of a hen's egg, have developed. The dried flowering tops were official in the *National Formulary* from 1916 to 1936.

THREE-LEAVED HOP TREE

The indigenous three-leaved hop tree sometimes called the wafer ash, was used by the Menominees as a sacred medicine. They mixed the root bark into other medicines to give them added potency.

It was introduced in the medical literature by Rafinesque in his work *Medical Botany* in 1830. He listed the leaves as being useful in the treatment of wounds and in the destruction of intestinal worms. Following this work and several others, the eclectic practitioners adopted wafer ash for a wide variety of problems.

It is included under "Sedatives" only because its common name suggests that it was regarded as being similar to the hop tree, which was an official sedative drug.

HOPS (FIG.88)

The use of hops in brewing beer is well known. What is little appreciated is the fact that the strobiles of this climbing species were used as sedatives both in Europe and America.

Hops are found wild and are indigenous to Europe, Asia, and North America; they were used as medicines in those three geographical regions. In 1787, when King George III was seriously ill, the court physicians filled his pillow with hops instead of opiates to calm his nerves and to promote sleep. In North America, the Indians discovered the value of hops independent of the Europeans. The Mohegans prepared a sedative medicine from the conelike strobiles and sometimes heated these pistillate blossoms and applied them for toothache.

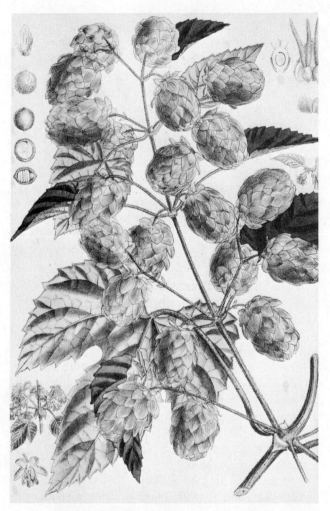

(FIG. 88) HOPS: *Several tribes used the strobiles of this well-known member of the hemp family as a sedative. The plant is also found in Europe, where the physicians to King George III filled his pillow with hops to calm his nerves and to induce sleep.*

One Meskwaki Indian practitioner cured insomnia with hops. The Dakota tribe utilized a tea of the steeped strobiles to relieve pains of the digestive organs, and the Menominee tribe regarded a related species of hops as a cure-all, a panacea.

Toward the close of the last century, hops were widely used in American medicine for their tonic, diuretic, and sedative properties. It was then held that hops exerted their calming effects on the heart as well as on the nervous system. The side effects described were colic and constipation.

The principal activity of hops is not in the conelike strobiles but in the glandular hairs of the fruiting body. These hairs contain lupulin, which is described as a sedative and hypnotic drug. This derivative was recognized in the *U.S. Pharmacopoeia* from 1831 through 1916.

Hops are used in brewing to add bitterness and to act as a preservative. This is the principal use of the plant, although at one time the young shoots were cooked and eaten as a substitute for asparagus. In Gerarde's herbal of 1633, it is written that, "The buds or first sprouts which come forth in the spring are used to be eaten in sallads; yet are they, as Pliny saith, more toothsome than nourishing, for they yield but very small nourishment." Only the young shoots are tasty, the older ones being so bitter and tough that some people bleached them with sulphuric oxide to soften them. King Henry VIII feared that he would be poisoned by this violent bleaching agent, an early food "softener," and he protected himself by passing an edict that forbade the addition of hops to ale brewed in his household.

As is the case with so many medicinally valuable plants, hops are also utilized for other useful purposes. The stems are made into a fiber while oil of hops is used in the manufacture of the fougrè or chypre-type perfumes.

Hops are widely cultivated, but have escaped and are found growing in thickets and along river banks where the plant thrives in the damp soil. The generic name *Humulus* is from *humus*, meaning earth. Because this vine tends to choke the plant on which it climbs, it was named *lupulus* for its wolflike habits. The English name *hop* is from the Anglo-Saxon *hoppan*, which means "to climb." It is easily recognized by its conelike strobiles, which are collected for brewing in September when the scales are gold in color. Interestingly, hops belongs to the hemp family, as does marijuana.

ᴈ WILD LETTUCE (FIG.89)

Varieties of wild lettuce which produce a milky juice similar in appearance and odor to opium have been used since antiquity to induce sleep and as sedatives. Whether this effect is real or imagined is still undergoing debate; however, it is known that the American Indians used lettuce plants in a number of remedies.

Meskwaki women imbibed a tea of prickly lettuce leaves after childbirth to promote the secretion of milk, while the Flambeau Ojibwas employed tall blue lettuce for the same purpose. The Menominees used the milky juice of wild lettuce on poison ivy rash.

Wild lettuce, indigenous to North America, was used in early American medicine for sedative purposes, especially in nervous complaints. The milky juice was also used to allay cough.

Lactuacarium, which is the dried milky juice of prickly lettuce and other species of lettuce, is used in medicines for its hypnotic, sedative, and diuretic properties. This substance is obtained when the tops of the stems are cut. A latex exudes which, like opium, is collected and dried in cups. Surprisingly, the active chemical constituents of these plants are not limited by the milky juice. Hyoscyamine, which is a powerful depressant of the parasympathetic nervous system that is similar in effect to that of belladonna and relatively abundant in jimson weed (*Datura stramonium*), is also found in two varieties of lettuce (*L. sativa* and *L. virosa* or prickly lettuce).

These facts are not included to create a run on the lettuce market and must be tempered by the remarks of physicians and pharmacologists who believe that any effects ascribed to these plants originate in the mind of the user. This superstition, they say, originated because of the similarity in appearance and scent between the latex of this species and the latex of the opium plant.

In any case, *lactuacarium* was official in the *U.S. Pharmacopoeia* from 1820 to 1926 and was used for its sedative and diuretic properties.

The wild lettuce that is illustrated is common to moist woods and clearings throughout North America. It shows a leafy stem from three to ten feet high and numerous small yellow flowers which appear between June and October. Although wild lettuce is of the same genus as garden lettuce, the only characteristics which they share are the milky juice and the leafy flowering stem.

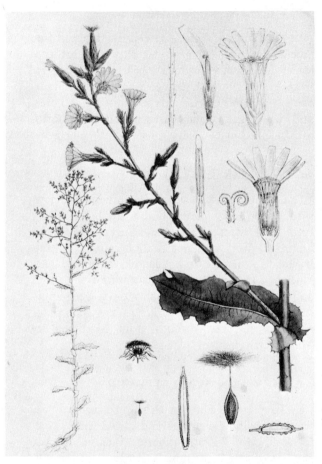

(FIG. 89) *WILD LETTUCE: Varieties of wild lettuce, which produce a milky juice similar in appearance and odor to opium, have been used since antiquity to induce sleep.*

SKIN PROBLEMS

Rashes and itching may be external manifestations of internal disorders. The American Indian treated these external disorders with many plants; a few of these, representing a wide geographical range, are listed below. The reader is also directed to specific categories of Indian treatment, as "Blisters," "Poison Ivy and Poison Oak," and "Boils." Although skin cancer and athlete's foot may not technically be considered skin problems, they are grouped in this category for convenience.

✤ WILD BERGAMOT

To dry up pimples the Winnebagos used the oil collected by boiling the leaves of wild bergamot. The Blackfoot Indians applied the boiled leaves directly on the pimples.

✤ WESTERN VIRGIN'S-BOWER

The Thompson Indians of British Columbia used a weak infusion of the whole western virgin's-bower as an external rinse for eczema and scabs. Also known as white clematis or traveler's joy, this climbing vine often chooses fences for support and bears numerous small white flowers, which are soon replaced by downy bunches of glistening fleece. This spectacle is beautiful to see, hence the name traveler's joy.

✤ WOOLY GROUNDSEL

The Hopis applied pulverized wooly groundsel leaves to pimples. The Zuñi treated aching bones with a wash made by steeping the pulverized roots of this plant. It is abundant in grassland areas, often growing where buffalo grass is found.

✤ YELLOW NUT GRASS

The Paiute Indians pounded the tubers of the perennial yellow nut grass together with tobacco leaves and applied the mass in a wet dressing to treat athlete's foot. This species is found in moist fields from southern Canada to Florida and Texas and also on the Pacific coast where it grows north to Alaska.

✤ NEW JERSEY TEA

During the American Revolution, the low shrub New Jersey tea was one of the main substitutes for Oriental tea and was in great demand. Since the plant does not contain caffeine, it was useless to some people but lauded by others. The Cherokee Indians used it as a wash for skin cancer and venereal sores. This plant is not geographically limited to the state of New Jersey. It is prevalent in dry, open woods from Manitoba to Maine, south to the Gulf of Mexico.

✤ WESTERN WALLFLOWER

To prevent sunburn the Zuñis applied the western wallflower ground and mixed with water. Generally, the Indians anointed themselves with the fats of various mammals and birds or fish oils to shield their skin from the sun's rays, but this plant application is one recorded exception. In Greek, *Erysimum*, the genus name, means "to draw blisters."

Many plants were employed to treat the itch; in California the Pomo boiled the bark of the willow common to their environment (*Salix lasiolepis*) and employed the liquid as a wash; the Potawatomis used a similar preparation but from the bark of the speckled alder; the Meskwakis similarly utilized white ash bark; and the Alabamas boiled the inner bark of the prickly ash.

SMALLPOX

WATER AVENS (FIG. 90)

The Thompson Indians of British Columbia reported that during a smallpox epidemic which occurred before 1900, every individual who drank a strong, dark decoction made from the boiled roots of a closely related species of avens survived the disease. They took the same preparation for any disease characterized by a rash, such as measles, chicken pox, etc. It was used by other tribes for sore throat and coughs.

The *Dispensatory of the United States* attributes the medicinal values of this species to the tannin it contains. This agent, valued for its property of drying out tissues, was used as an astringent when it was official in the *U.S. Pharmacopoeia* from 1820 to 1882

The water avens is found in meadows and bogs throughout Canada and the northern states. The boiled root was once known as Indian chocolate and was drunk with sugar and milk. The plant is used as a chocolate substitute throughout the year, but one expert on wild foods thinks it is at its best in the fall or early spring. This beverage was formerly valued as a tasty home remedy for dysentery, diarrhea, and stomach upsets. Since the drink is said to be delicious and does contain tannin, this may have been one of our earliest "sugar-coated medicines."

PITCHER PLANT (FIG. 91)

The swamp dwelling pitcher plant was once regarded as being a specific cure for smallpox by many tribes of Canada and the Great Lakes region of the United States. The Indians believed that the use of the root not only offered some form of immunity but shortened the term of the disease when contracted and prevented the formation of deep "pits" in convalescence.

(FIG. 90) WATER AVENS: *The Thompson Indians claimed that every individual who drank a strong tea of these roots survived a smallpox epidemic which took the lives of hundreds.*

(FIG. 91) PITCHER PLANT: *Many Canadian tribes believed that the use of these roots offered some immunity from smallpox or prevented the formation of deep scars occurring in convalescence.*

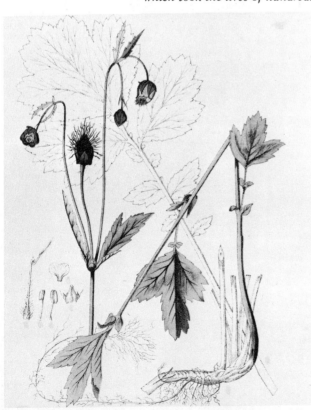

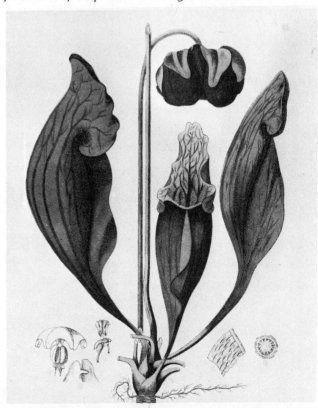

A British surgeon corroborated the Indians' view with regard to the effectiveness of pitcher plant when in 1861, he delivered a paper in London citing his experiences in Canada. During a smallpox epidemic among the Indians, *every* case was cured by an infusion of the root as administered by an old Indian woman.

Nevertheless the physicians of that time did not accept the pitcher plant into their practices, nor was it accepted in the pharmacopoeias. Dr. Millspaugh cites a reference he found scrawled

across the face of an article on the use of this drug in small-pox. . . . A former owner of the book has written: This medicine was thoroughly tested by Mr. John Thomas Lane in the spring of 1864 at the Small-pox Hospital at Claremont, in Alexandria, Va., for the period of several weeks, in the presence of the medical officers of the Third Division Hospital; and proved to be without any curative powers in this disease, and Mr. Lane a humbug. He lost more than fifty per cent of the cases of variola committed to him, more than were lost by any other treatment.

The same author then cites examples of men who were equally confident that an infusion of the root was absolutely beneficial in smallpox, one man declaring that his brother's life was saved by this remedy!

Here then is another example of a plant remedy that was highly regarded by the Indians and rejected by official medical circles. Might this prove to be a plant worthy of further research?

CARMINE THISTLE

The Navajos of Arizona and Utah prepared a lotion of the entire carmine thistle plant and chewed the freshly dug root to treat smallpox. This distinctive species was also used in most cases of fever. This plant belongs to a genus that contains many edible species.

SNAKEBITE

One medical expert states that the Indians were considerably skilled in treating snakebite. Treatment was generally initiated with an incision of the bite, which was followed by suction. Some practitioners then applied a part of the snake to the wound as a kind of ritualistic offering, while others applied various plants, several of which are described below.

Dr. Eric Stone also discusses other aspects of snakebite treatment among the Indians:

> It is probable that the tribes of the Southwest which practiced the Snake Dance knew something, empirically if not theoretically, about immunization. In the ceremony the participants allowed themselves to be bitten by full-grown rattlesnakes, yet suffered no ill effects. As neophytes in the order, they had desensitized themselves by first submitting to the bite of young snakes with weak virus, gradually increasing the age of the snakes until they could receive the bite of the adult with impunity.

Some of the drugs used on the wounds include the following.

✍ PURPLE CONEFLOWER

Purple coneflower species was a panacea among many Plains tribes. The Missouri River tribes employed it as an antidote for snakebites and for the stings and bites of insects. A piece of the plant was also used for toothache and mumps. The same tribes commonly washed their hands in a decoction of the plant to enable them to withstand heat. The Sioux drank a decoction of the root as a remedy for hydrophobia and snakebites.

This perennial herb was used in American medicine to induce profuse sweating and was official in the *National Formulary* from 1916 to 1950.

✍ SENECA SNAKEROOT (FIG.92)

The interesting history of the Seneca snakeroot, from the time it was first noticed by a Scot physician as it was used by the Seneca Indians for

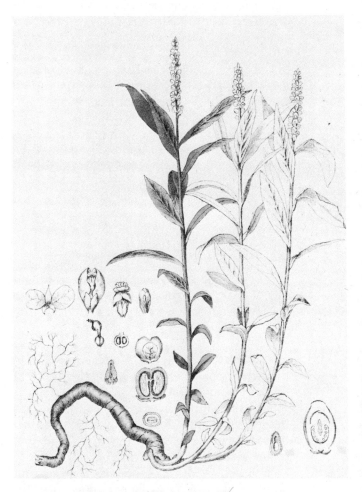

(FIG. 92) SENECA SNAKEROOT: *The Senecas chewed the roots of this plant and applied them as a wet mash to snakebites.*

snakebite to its adoption in the treatment of coughs and other respiratory troubles, is traced elsewhere in this book (see "Coughs").

As with most snakebite remedies, the roots of this species were chewed and then applied directly on the bite.

Since the twisted root could easily represent a snake, it is not difficult to imagine how the first Seneca Indian "discovered" this remedy.

Seneca snakeroot contains senegin, which is a saponinlike compound, and polygalic acid. It was official in the *U.S. Pharmacopoeia* from 1820 to 1936 and was used as a stimulant and as an expectorant.

Button snakeroot was often substituted for Seneca snakeroot and was described by an early writer on American medicinal plants as being similar in action. This species was accepted as an official medicine, and surprisingly, it too was employed to promote perspiration and for respiratory congestion.

This member of the milkwort family inhabits rocky woods and hillsides throughout the eastern states. The knobby-topped root sends up fifteen to twenty or more slender stems, which are from six inches to a foot in height. The small, greenish white flowers which are borne on the ends of the stems, bloom between May and June. The twisted root was collected in the fall and brought a high price of from fifty-five to seventy cents a pound around 1909.

✑ VIRGINIA SNAKEROOT (FIG.93)

The Virginia snakeroot is the most famous Indian snakebite remedy. Its repute spread so quickly that it was utilized in England and admitted to the London *Pharmacopoeia* as early as 1650.

This is a strange genus of plants, for as Dr. Millspaugh pointed out, "almost all the species of this large genus are esteemed, by the natives of the countries in which they grow, as remedies against the poisonous effects of snake bites . . . this use being fully known to each nation without previous communication with each other."

Naturally, as with most popular remedies, this plant was used for many illnesses other than the one for which it was originally recognized. It was accepted in the *U.S. Pharmacopoeia* and employed for tonic and stimulant purposes. It contains borneal, which is a volatile oil; aristolochine, an alkaloid; and other, less important, constituents. The alkaloidal principle has reportedly produced respiratory paralysis.

In general, the Indians simply chewed the root and applied it to snakebite. Over one hundred

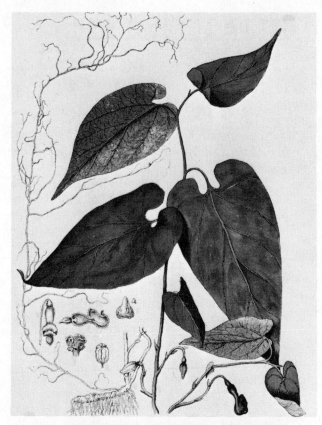

(FIG. 93) *VIRGINIA SNAKEROOT: This plant is the most famous Indian snakebite remedy. Its reputation spread so quickly that it was included in the* London Pharmacopoeia *as early as 1650.*

years ago this was the most highly prized snakebite remedy of all and was often carried in the packs of woodsmen.

This plant is basically restricted to woods from Michigan to Connecticut and extends south through the Allegheny Mountains. The wavy stem grows between one and three feet in height, and the solitary purple flower appears about July. When used in medicine, the roots were collected in the fall.

If a Hopi was bitten by a snake he chewed the root of bladderpod and applied it on the wound, while the Winnebago and Dakota Indians boiled the buds of white ash and drank the resulting tea to offset the poison.

SORE THROAT

Many remedies appear in the literature to treat the common sore throat. As is the case with diarrhea or dysentery, the Indians employed many different plants which appear to have astringent properties. Some of these are listed below.

BARBERRY (FIG. 94)

Soon after the barberry's introduction to America, this European relative of the Oregon grape was employed by several tribes for medicinal

(FIG. 94) *BARBERRY: The Penobscots of Maine applied the mashed roots or bark to mouth ulcers or sore throats.*

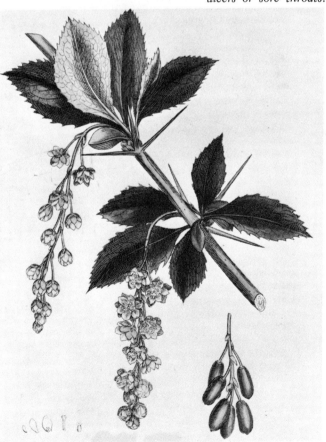

purposes. The Penobscots of Maine applied the mashed roots or bark to mouth ulcers or sore throat. The Catawabas used a stem or root infusion for stomach ulcers. Since the barberry was employed in Europe for similar purposes, it is safe to assume that the Indians borrowed the uses for this species from the early settlers.

BLOODROOT

To cure sore throat, the Pillager Ojibwas squeezed the root juices of bloodroot on a piece of maple sugar and held the astringent lump in their mouths.

SLIPPERY ELM

The Pillager Ojibwas treated sore throat with a tea made from the inner bark of slippery elm.

GOLDENROD

The Zuñi chewed goldenrod blossoms and slowly swallowed the juice to cure sore throat.

WHITE PINE

Young, green needles of the white pine were boiled and the resulting tea drunk by various northern tribes.

SENNA (American)

Although the senna is today most frequently employed for its laxative effects, the seeds were soaked in water and swallowed by the Meskwaki to cure sore throat.

SPRUCE

The Crees ate the small cones of spruce trees to treat sore throat.

STAGHORN SUMAC

A tea of staghorn sumac berries was taken by the Micmacs for sore throat. A sore-throat gargle that was prepared from a related species, smooth upland sumac, was once commonly prescribed by country doctors.

YAMPA

In the Northwest, the Blackfoot Indians chewed the root of yampa and slowly swallowed the juice to relieve sore throat.

THRUSH

The Indian practitioner probably distinguished the thrush mouth infection from common mouth sores and ulcers by the characteristic white patches commonly associated with thrush. Although goldthread was the most popular plant remedy for common mouth sores among both Indians and the early settlers, it was probably also used in treating thrush in children. Since this plant has been discussed elsewhere, it is not included in this section.

❧ GERANIUM

The Cherokees boiled geranium root together with wild grape, and with the liquid, rinsed the mouths of children affected with thrush. Geranium was also used by the Pillager Ojibwas to treat mouth ulcers.

This became a popular domestic remedy, and geranium is described as being an effective astringent that is useful in sore throat and mouth ulcers in the 23d edition of the *Dispensatory of the United States*. The rhizome of this species was official in the *U.S. Pharmacopoeia* from 1820 to 1916 when it was used for its astringent properties.

Geranium, one of the most common native wild flowers, grows in clearings and open woods. Its hairy stem grows between one and two feet high and from April to June bears purple flowers. As with most botanicals collected for medicinal purposes, the roots are gathered in the fall when they are rich with constituents for the coming winter.

❧ PERSIMMON

Famous for its delicious fruits to those who live within the range of its growth, the persimmon was used by the Catawba Indians to cure thrush. They stripped the bark from the tree and boiled it in water, utilizing the resulting dark liquid as a mouth rinse.

Persimmon was utilized in American medicine for its value as an astringent, and was an official drug in the *U.S. Pharmacopoeia* from 1880 to 1882. The leaves, said to be high in vitamin C, are eaten by some people to prevent scurvy.

❧ RATTLESNAKE PLANTAIN

The rattlesnake plantain herb, common to dry woods in the eastern United States, was favored by the Mohegans, who applied the mashed leaves to prevent thrush in infants.

TOOTHACHE

⅍ PRICKLY ASH (FIG. 95)

Before describing the Indian uses for the prickly ash species, I would like to include Dr. Millspaugh's observations concerning the use of prickly ash bark as a remedy for toothache:

> From personal experience one day in the woods while botanizing, I found that, upon chewing the bark for relief of toothache, speedy mitigation of the pain followed, though the sensation of the acrid bark was nearly or fully as unpleasant as the ache, and so painful finally in itself that I abandoned its use, only to have the toothache return when the irritation of the bark had left the mucous membranes.

The Houma Indians employed the pulverized roots and bark for toothache, while the Alabama tribe used only the roots for this complaint. Usage of this species is reported among many tribes—the Ojibwas, Menominees, Meskwakis, and Comanches all utilized the plant in various ways.

Several species were employed in domestic American medicine for toothache, in rheumatism, and as an external counterirritant. The southern variety was once known as toothache tree. Both the dried bark and berries have been official in the *U.S. Pharmacopoeia.*

The genus name, *Zanthoxylum,* is derived from two Greek words which refer to the yellow color of the roots. The specific name for southern prickly ash, *Clava-Herculis,* means "club of Hercules," which refers to the large corky excrescences growing on the bark.

Both species are indigenous to the United States and belong to the rue family. The southern variety seldom grows above four to five feet in height and is sometimes only a shrub. The trunk shows gray bark with sharp spines or prickles, a characteristic of this species. Numerous small greenish white flowers appear about June. These are followed by black berries, which contain wrinkled seeds.

The northern variety (Z. *americanum*), which

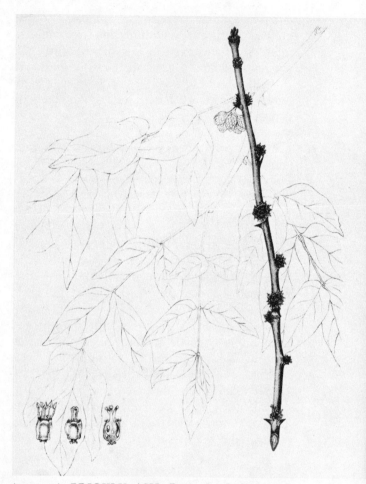

(FIG. 95) *PRICKLY ASH: Both the Indians and the whites chewed the bark for relief of toothache.*

is covered with sharp, scattered prickles, grows from about four to twenty-five feet in height. The flowers are small and green and are found near the origin of the new shoots. It has alternate, pinnate leaves, each one consisting of four or five leaflets in pairs. Oval capsules appear which are greenish red in color. It can be found in damp woods and other damp, shady areas from Quebec to Virginia and west to Ontario, South Dakota, through Kansas and Nebraska. The odor of the leaves resembles that of lemon oil. The flowers appear before the foliage, in the early spring.

Many other plants were utilized in Indian medicine to alleviate toothache; those which follow are easy to recognize. The Minok tribe of California chewed the stalks of the gold-back fern, while the Pimas heated the tips of branches of the creosote bush and dripped the sap into the offending cavity. The Alabamas inserted a small piece of goldenrod root into cavities.

Plains tribes were said to have chewed the rootstock of sweet flag, while the Meskwakis applied root hairs or rootlets of skunk cabbage to affected teeth. Finally, we come to see another application of that much-used plant, the common geranium. The Meskwaki Indians, originally of the Wisconsin region, boiled the roots and rinsed their mouths with the solution for toothache, sore gums, and pyorrhea.

VENEREAL DISEASES

It is generally believed that syphilis and gonorrhea were introduced to North America by the Europeans. Early American doctors generally agreed that venereal diseases were unknown in pre-Columbian times. As you may imagine, the Indian was usually bewildered by these diseases, and he usually treated only the visible sores and rashes. Unaware of the systemic nature of these diseases, he resorted to many different plant remedies, some of which are enumerated below. The records also show other treatments. For example, the Crow practitioners had the patient squat, bringing the genitals into close proximity with rocks which were heated in a fire.

In reviewing the following plant remedies which were used by various Indian tribes, it is well to remember that gonorrhea is an inflammation of the mucous membranes of the genitals and that this disease is caused by the gonococcus bacteria *Neisseria gonorrhoeae*. Syphilis is a chronic venereal disease that is characterized by a lesion which appears two to four weeks after contact, and which changes from a small red swelling to an ulcer to a hardened chancre. It is transmitted by direct contact between people or by contact with contaminated objects or by the transfusion of infected blood or in the birth canal from an infected mother to the fetus. The spirochete which causes syphilis, *Treponema pallidum*, may enter the body through any break in the skin or mucous membrane. If any of these remedies were effective (and this is impossible for us to decide), the plants would have had to contain specific antibacterial properties.

⤐ PRICKLY ASH

The bark and roots of prickly ash were boiled in fresh water and about one pint of the decoction was taken in a single dose. An interesting record of the use of this plant by a Winnebago chief who cured a white trader of gonorrhea around 1766 is found in J. Carver's *Travels through the Interior Parts of North America*.

The dried bark of this species was official in the *U.S. Pharmacopoeia* from 1820 to 1926, when it was used to treat rheumatic complaints. The berries, used for antispasmodic, stimulant, and antirheumatic purposes, were listed in the *National Formulary* from 1916 to 1947.

The *Dispensatory of the United States* notes that several species contain berberine which may be a mild sedative. Perhaps for this reason the plant was also used to treat toothache by the Houmas, who inserted the ground bark and roots into cavities; by the Alabamas, who used the scraped roots on aching teeth; and by the Comanches, who also used the bark to treat toothache.

A related species found in the south, southern prickly ash, is also known by the name toothache tree. Another relative, *Zanthoxylum macrophyllum*, is used in Africa to treat toothache.

⤐ LONGLEAF EPHEDRA

The dried, crushed longleaf ephedra was applied externally to syphilitic sores by the Navajos. The Hopis drank a tea from the branches and twigs of a related species to treat the same disease.

⤐ BALSAM FIR

The Ojibwas made a warm liquid of the gummy sap of balsam fir and drank it freely to cure gonorrhea.

⤐ OREGON GRAPE

The Klikata tribe drank strong doses of boiled root decoctions of the Oregon grape. The roots, which contain berberine and three other alkaloids, were official in the *U.S. Pharmacopoeia* from 1905 to 1916 when they were used as a bitter tonic.

✑ ROCKY MOUNTAIN JUNIPER

The Paiute Indians drank a tea of the terminal twigs of Rocky Mountain juniper in the treatment of syphilis.

✑ GREAT LOBELIA (FIG.96)

The scientific name of the great lobelia, *siphilitica*, indicates that it was widely used to treat this disease. The Iroquois in the Mohawk Valley of New York used a root decoction to treat syphilis as did English physicians of the early 1800s. Dr. Millspaugh offers an interesting theory as to why the plant failed to effect a cure when employed in Europe:

The natives of North America are said to have held this plant a secret in the cure of syphilis, until it was purchased from them . . . and intro-

(FIG. 96) GREAT LOBELIA: *The Iroquois attempted to treat venereal disease with a strong tea made of these roots. Although it was widely held that this remedy effectively cured the ulcers among the Indians, the same remedy effected no change in patients when used in Europe.*

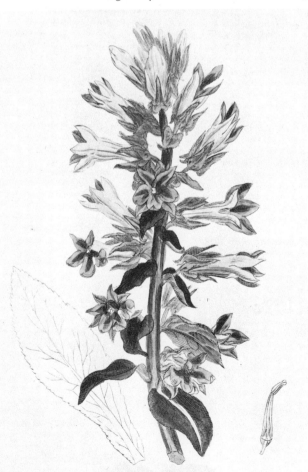

duced . . . as a drug of great repute in that disease. European physicians, however, failed to cure with it, and finally cast it aside, though Linnaeus, thinking it justified its Indian reputation, gave the species its distinctive name, *syphilitica*. The cause of failure may be the fact that the aborigines did not trust to the plant alone, but always used it in combination with may-apple roots (*Podophyllum peltatum*), the bark of the wild cherry (*Prunus Virginica*), and dusted the ulcers with the powdered bark of New Jersey tea (*Ceanothus Americanus*). Another chance of failure lay in the volatility of its active principle, as the dried herb was used.

✑ PINE

The Fox and Chippewa boiled the inner bark of pine and drank large quantities of the resulting liquid to cure gonorrhea.

✑ WILD ROSE

The Mescalero Apaches boiled wild rosebuds and imbibed the resulting tea to cure gonorrhea.

✑ SLENDERLEAF SKELETON PLANT

A decoction of the whole slenderleaf skeleton plant was drunk by tribes of the Southwest in the treatment of syphilis.

✑ SUMAC (FIG.97)

Either the smooth upland sumac or the mountain sumac was used to treat the external sores of gonorrhea by the Chippewas of Minnesota and the Thompsons of British Columbia. Although it is not clear which plant was employed, the preparation consisted of the boiled stems and roots in water. About one pint of the decoction was taken in a single dose; this was often not repeated through the course of the disease. The Thompsons were aware of the dangerous properties of these species, and they considered this remedy poisonous in large dosages.

The use of mountain sumac by the American Indians was noted in 1806 in the *Journals of the Lewis and Clark Expedition*:

The Chippaways use a decoction of the root . . . of a species of Sumac common to the Atlantic

States and to this country near and on the western side of the Rocky Mountains. . . . These decoctions are drank freely and without limitation. The same decoctions are used also in cases of the Gonnarea and are effecatious and sovereign. Notwithstanding that this disorder does exist among the indians on the Columbia yet it is witnessed in but few individuals, high up the river, or at least the males who are always sufficiently exposed to the observation or inspection of the phisician. In my whole rout down this river I did not see more than two or three with Gonnarea and about double that number with the pox.

Mountain sumac is easily distinguished from other sumacs by the winged shape of its leaf stalk between the leaflets.

✑§ THISTLE

The Zuñis steeped the whole thistle plant overnight in cold water and drank the infusion three times daily. Men were required to run after each dose of the medicine to encourage sweating and they were then wrapped in blankets. This treatment often caused nausea and vomiting.

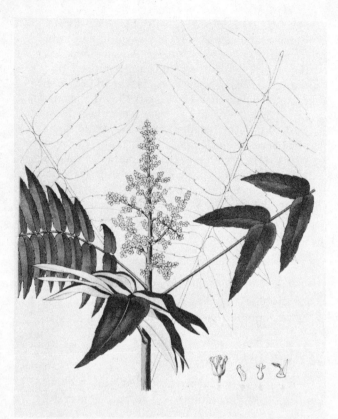

(FIG. 97) SMOOTH UPLAND SUMAC: *Several tribes treated the external sores of gonorrhea with a wash of the roots and stems of the sumacs.*

VOMITING

Without looking for causes, the native American usually treated the symptoms of illnesses. Nausea and vomiting, when not self-induced prior to ceremonies, were treated with various plant preparations.

✑ SHARP-LEAVED BEARDTONGUE

The leaves of the perennial sharp-leaved beardtongue were steeped in warm water by the Blackfoot Indians who drank the resulting tea to stop vomiting.

✑ LOW RUNNING BLACKBERRY

To arrest violent vomiting, the Kwakiutls of Vancouver Island, British Columbia, boiled the peeled roots and vines of low running blackberry together with thimbleberry and drank the astringent liquid.

✑ ROCKY MOUNTAIN MAPLE

The Thompson Indians of British Columbia drank a decoction of boiled Rocky Mountain maple bark and wood to cure nausea, especially when it was brought about by the odor of a corpse.

This is a small shrub or tree seldom growing above thirty-five feet in height. Its leaves have three to five lobes and senate edges. The flowers are yellowish green, and the typical maple "wings" are between four and six inches wide. This short maple is found near streams and on hillsides throughout the Rocky Mountain region —north to Montana and south to Arizona.

✑ WILD MINT

The Cheyennes prepared a decoction of the ground leaves and stems of wild mint and drank the liquid to check nausea. Pulegone and thymol are derived from an oil of wild mint.

This is the only native species of mint in America, spearmint and peppermint having been naturalized from Europe. Wild mint is easily distinguished from the other mints by its whorled flowers which are borne in the axils of the leaves. The other species of mint bear their flowers in the upper portion of their stems. Its odor resembles that of peppermint. The species is common on stream banks throughout America. (The leaves make an excellent tea.)

In their part of the country, the Penobscots prepared a tea of alder bark to alleviate nausea and vomiting, while in the region of the Mississippi–Louisiana boundary, the Houma tribe prepared a decoction of the boiled roots of ginseng.

Self-induced vomiting on a daily basis was frequently practiced in many tribes. This was considered to be a purifying experience and also a means of obtaining strength prior to a hunting or war expedition. To accomplish this, mechanical means were employed (a feather tickling the back of the throat) as were other nonbotanical methods, such as the ingestion of large quantities of warm, salty water.

WARTS

◆§ PRICKLY PEAR CACTUS (FIG.98)

Many members of the genus of cactus to which prickly pear cactus belongs served as important food sources for numerous American Indians; they were not frequently employed as medicines. However, one detailed record on the Blackfoot tribe states that these Indians removed warts and moles by lacerating their swellings and then applying the "fuzz" from this variety. The same tribe bound peeled stems of this same species on wounds as a dressing. The fresh flowers and green ovaries were used to some extent by physicians of the late nineteenth century. They also employed a drink made of the cactus joints boiled in water for pulmonary complaints and applied the same part, baked, to fresh wounds.

This species inhabits rocky places and sandy areas of both coasts as well as the dry plains of the Southwest. It bears light yellow flowers from May through June.

Various species of milkweed (FIG.99) were employed by the Catawba Indians who rubbed the milky juice of the plants directly on warts. Although the May apple was primarily used for its laxative effects, the Penobscot tribe applied the crushed root to warts. Finally, although there is no record of Indian usage, the juice of celandine was once popularly applied to warts and corns in American domestic medicine. This plant belongs to the poppy family, contains five to seven alkaloids, and was used for its sedative and cathartic action when it was official in the U.S. Pharmacopoeia. Naturalized from Europe, celandine frequents rich, wet soil along roadsides and fences in the northeastern United States and southern Canada. It is easily recognized by its small, sulphur yellow flowers which bloom from about April to September and by a milky orange juice on the stem.

(FIG. 98) PRICKLY PEAR CACTUS: *The Blackfeet treated warts by lacerating them and applying the fuzz from this cactus.*

(FIG. 99) MILKWEED: *The Catawba Indians rubbed the milky juice of the milkweeds on warts.*

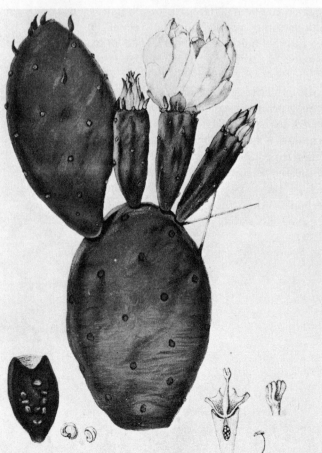

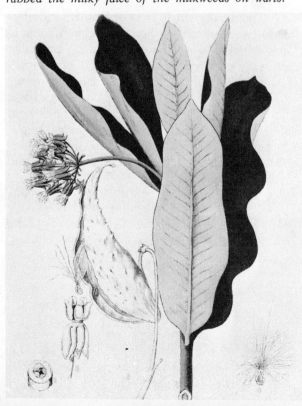

WHOOPING COUGH

~§ AMERICAN CHESTNUT (FIG.100)

The American chestnut is the only plant that is reported to have been used by an Indian tribe against whooping cough. It appears as if the Mohegans learned to use a tea of the leaves against this infectious coughing disease from the whites, who derived the remedy from an unknown source. Although Dr. Millspaugh wrote that chestnut leaves were used for whooping cough and it was then thought that they effected a "sedative action on the nerves of respiration," the *Dispensatory of the United States* of 1942 called this belief a superstition, adding, "there is . . . no sufficient reason to believe them to possess any therapeutic value except that of a mild astringent." For this purpose the leaves were official in the U.S. *Pharmacopoeia* from 1873 to 1905. The dried leaves contain 9 percent tannic acid; they were gathered in the early fall and used for their astringent properties.

Despite its apparent lack of medicinal value, the chestnut tree is highly esteemed for its edible nuts and will be discussed in greater detail under "Earth Foods." This native variety rarely grows higher than eighty feet nor does the trunk often exceed a diameter of four feet. Exceptions do exist—in the late 1800s, one specimen in New York Harbor was thought to be five hundred years old and was so large that it was then popularly called the elephant. An exceptionally broad chestnut tree, measuring twenty-two feet in diameter, was recorded near Seymour, Indiana, in 1880.

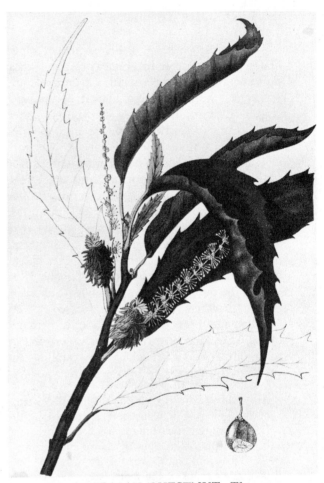

(FIG. 100) AMERICAN CHESTNUT: *The Mohegans learned to use a tea made from the leaves to treat whooping cough, caught from the white settlers.*

WORMS

✑ PINKROOT (FIG. 101)

The pinkroot is one of the clearest examples of acceptance of an Indian remedy by the medical profession. The Cherokees called it *unsteetla* and prepared a worm medicine from it by boiling a large quantity of the freshly dug root in water. In the early 1700s, two physicians from Charleston, South Carolina, learned about pinkroot's efficacy from the Indians. The word soon spread to the general public, who praised this worm treatment, particularly against roundworms, for the next two hundred years. Pinkroot fell into disuse in the early 1900s simply because greedy herb dealers adulterated or even substituted shipments of true pinkroot with quantities of other plants, notably the East Tennessee pinkroot. Even though the public needs drugs which are effective, it soon abandoned what has been called "a very excellent and useful drug." I cite a letter from one of the Charleston physicians, Dr. Garden, written to a colleague in England in 1763 extolling the virtues of this species:

> About forty years ago, the antihelminthic virtues of the root of this plant were discovered by the Indians; since which time it has been much used here by physicians, practitioners, and planters. . . . To a child of two years of age, who had been taking ten grains of the root twice a day, without having any other effect than making her dull and giddy, I prescribed twenty-two grains morning and evening which purged her briskly, and brought away five large worms.

In actual practice, the fresh root was preferred; one medical text cautions against using pinkroot stored longer than two years. The 23d edition of the *Dispensatory of the United States* lists the prescribed dose of the powdered root for an adult as four or eight grams each morning and evening for several days, this sequence then to be followed by a strong laxative.

Although it was once abundant in the South, pinkroot may today be rare in its native environ-

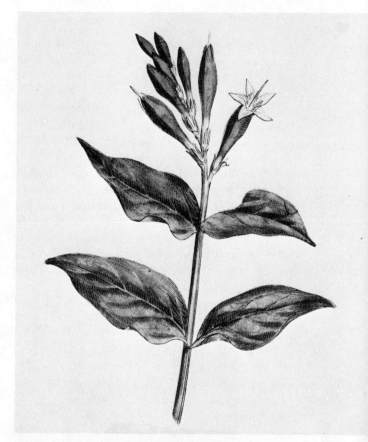

(FIG. 101) PINKROOT: *The Cherokees made a worm medicine by boiling a large quantity of the fresh root in water. News of its success soon spread among the whites who employed this worm treatment for the next two hundred years.*

ment, mainly the deep woods from New Jersey to Florida.

This member of the logania family (which contains many poisonous species) appears as a single erect stem from six to eighteen inches high, with pairs of broad lance-shaped stalkless leaves from two to four inches long. The brilliant trumpet-shaped flowers, which appear from May to July, are bright red on the outside and yellow within. The small rootstock, which is collected in the fall, has an aromatic odor and a bitter, pungent taste.

PUMPKIN (FIG. 102)

Another plant employed against worms is the pumpkin. Although it was *not* used by the Indians for this purpose (some tribes used the crushed seeds on wounds, others employed an infusion of the seeds as a diuretic, etc.), a popular American home remedy for worms consisted of a tea made of pumpkin seed.

TULIP TREE

The stately tulip tree was only casually employed against worms by the Indians. The Catawba tribe ingested the root bark to expel worms, while the seeds were given to Indian children of the West for the same purpose. This plant has since been employed in domestic medicine to reduce fever and to increase the urine flow. The bark of this tree was official in the *U.S. Pharmacopoeia* from 1820 to 1882, when it was utilized for its tonic and diuretic properties.

The inner bark of the tulip poplar contains tulipiferine, which reportedly exerts powerful effects on the heart and nervous system. The *Dispensatory of the United States* says that the powdered bark has been used for rheumatism and digestive problems.

The light yellow to brown wood has been used in cabinet work and as shingles.

WORMSEED

Wormseed is another example of a once-popular and reputedly effective worm medicine that has since been replaced by synthetic agents. It is not clear how the Indians came to recognize the value of this species, but it is certain that several tribes were using it before the coming of the European.

The American Indian may have learned about wormseed from a Mexican or South American counterpart. This could have occurred at the time of the Spanish conquests in Mexico which forced many Mexican Indians to flee northward to escape the vicious gold-seeking conquistadors. R. L. Roys in his *Ethno-Botany of the Maya* believes that wormseed was utilized to expel worms by practitioners of that civilization. Indigenous to Mexico and South America, wormseed became naturalized as far north as New England as its reputation as a vermifuge spread.

Whereas the Natchez Indians employed an

(FIG. 102) PUMPKIN: *A popular American home remedy for worms consisted of a tea made of pumpkinseed.*

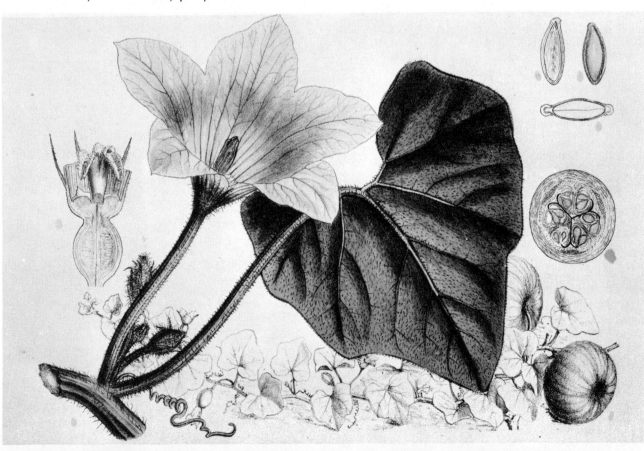

undisclosed part of the plant as a method of expelling worms in children, American physicians of the late 1800s recommended three to ten drops of expressed wormseed oil on sugar three times a day for several days, followed by a strong laxative. At that time it was considered to be especially effective against roundworms and was as popular as a home remedy as it was in medical circles.

The oil of chenopodium, which is derived from the seeds and other overground parts, was official in the *U.S. Pharmacopoeia* from 1820 to 1947 and in the *National Formulary* from 1947 to 1960. It has found its widest application as an effective agent against roundworms, hookworms, and other intestinal parasites, while it is said to be less effective against tapeworms. This is not a "safe" drug, in that poisoning and death have resulted from as small a dose as four drops three times a day for two days given to a one-year-old baby. Other deaths resulting from oil of chenopodium have been reported, and it has been established that fasting should *not* precede its use.

Wormseed, which occurs in waste places throughout North America, has a many-branched stem about two to three feet high and oblong or lancelike leaves. The lower leaves are one to five inches long, the upper leaves being much smaller. The small greenish flowers appear from July to September and are followed by small green fruits.

Of lesser renown as vermifuges were the wild plum (the Ojibwas drank a tea of the roots), American hemp (the Penobscots drank a root tea of it and named the plant worm root), and the running swamp blackberry. Although the blackberry was primarily utilized as a diarrhea remedy, the Mohegans drank infusions of the berries steeped in warm water to rid themselves of worms. The same tribe made a worm medicine from spearmint or peppermint, the leaves of the latter plant also being employed as a tea to rid babies of intestinal parasites.

WOUNDS

Perhaps it was due to their vigorous life styles that the native inhabitants of North America were early experts in the treatment of wounds. Without laboratories for chemical analysis, many herbs with antiseptic properties were discovered and utilized in Indian medicine. One writer on this subject thought that the Indians became skillful in finding and using these treatments because of the frequency with which wounds occurred and the necessity for treating them. Dr. Eric Stone, who was impressed with the Indians' ability to withstand serious wounds, wrote:

Suffice it, that all military and medical observers who came in contact with the Indians agree that they recovered more rapidly than the white from most wounds, and many recovered from wounds which would have been fatal to the white man. Bourke reports the cases of two Indians who were discharged from a military hospital that they might die among their people, yet made rapid recoveries as soon as their own medicine-men began their treatment. At a time when gunshot wounds of the bladder were invariably fatal to the white, the Indians seemed to suffer this accident with impunity. Loskiel examined a man whose face had been torn away, his rib cage crushed, limbs ripped and the abdomen disemboweled by a bear, yet had been able to crawl four miles to his village and in six months had completely recovered, except for extensive scarring. Such records could be continued almost indefinitely as all observers were so impressed by this ability to survive terrific wounds that hundreds have been reported.

Some of the botanical remedies employed for wounds are enumerated below.

ANEMONE

The root of the erect, perennial herb anemone was one of the most highly prized wound medicines of the Omaha and the Ponca tribes. A wash was prepared from the pounded boiled root and applied externally to the point of injury.

Anemonin, which is found in many related species of anemone, is clinically asserted to be a potent antiseptic substance.

ALUMROOT

The large woody alumroot was powdered by the Meskwakis and other tribes and applied to cuts, wounds, and skin sores that would not heal. The dried rhizomes and roots were utilized for the same purposes by the whites when these plant parts were officially accepted in the U.S. *Pharmacopoeia* between 1880 and 1882.

BLUE FLAG (FIG.103)

The blue flag species was one of the most popular of all American Indian medicines. The Penobscots valued it for treating most ailments, while other tribes assigned more specific roles to this member of the iris family. To relieve the swelling and pain associated with sores and bruises, the root was boiled in water and then pounded between stones. The pulped root mass was applied in a wet dressing and the affected part rinsed with the water in which the root was boiled. As a variation on this treatment, the Tadoussac tribe of Quebec combined the whole crushed plant with flour and applied the mixture as a poultice for bodily pain.

Surprisingly, blue flag was not employed for the above purposes by the general medical practitioners of the United States. It became an official drug and was entered in the U.S. *Pharmacopoeia* from 1820 through 1895 when it was utilized as an agent to induce vomiting or to promote drastic purging of the bowels. It was also used to promote the collection and excretion of excess bodily fluids.

The generic name, *Iris*, is derived from the Greek word for rainbow, while its specific name, *versicolor*, means "to change color" in Latin. The blue flag iris can be found in wet meadows, marshes, and damp meadows from Newfoundland to Manitoba south to Arkansas and Florida. The

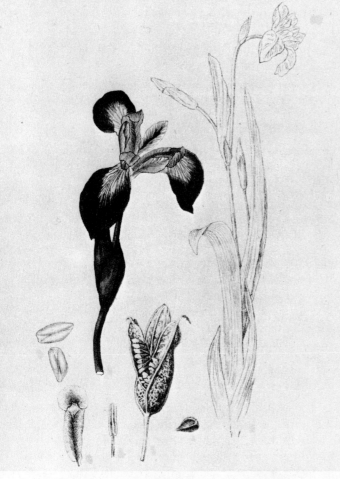

(FIG. 103) *BLUE FLAG: To relieve the swelling and pain associated with sores and bruises, many tribes applied the crushed bulb of this iris.*

violet blue flowers are veined with yellow, green, and white and are usually in bloom from May through July.

⊷ CHAIN FERN

The Luiseño tribe of southern California steeped chain fern roots in water and utilized the resulting liquid to alleviate the pains of wounds and bruises.

⊷ CLUB MOSS (FIG.104)

The yellowish spores of club moss were dusted on wounds or inhaled to stop nosebleed by the Blackfoot and Potawatomi tribes. They were official in the *U.S. Pharmacopoeia* from 1863 to 1947 when they were used to absorb fluids from injured tissue. The spores were formerly used in making theatrical explosives and lighting stages,

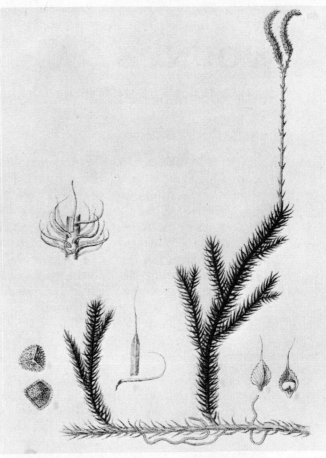

(FIG. 104) *CLUB MOSS: The Blackfeet dusted the yellowish spores of this moss on wounds to stop bleeding.*

as well as medicinally to prevent pills from sticking to one another in closed containers.

⊷ DEATH CAMASS

The Blackfoot Indians alleviated the pain of sprains and bruises by applying a wet, bound dressing of the pulped bulbs of the poisonous death camass to affected parts.

⊷ FIVE-FINGER FERN

Indians of the northwestern United States sometimes carried the five-finger fern on war expeditions as an agent in their *materia medica*. The fronds were chewed and applied to wounds to stop bleeding.

⊷ WILD GERANIUM

The perennial wild geranium was a favorite remedy of the Indians who lived on Great Manitoulin Island in Lake Huron. They applied the dried, powdered root on bleeding blood vessels to promote coagulation. Clinical experiments with rabbits have shown that it causes an increase in the clotting of blood, due primarily to the tannin contained in geranium.

☙ OREGON ASH

The Yokia tribe of Mendocino County pulverized the fresh roots of the Oregon ash and applied the mash to cure all serious wounds.

An interesting tale of a bear fight ends with a description of this Indian cure used to treat the deep wounds suffered in the battle. As described by V. K. Chestnut, the bear was finally felled with a club of mountain mahogany:

> One old Indian related a story about a bear fight which he had seen his father, a very powerful man, engage in when he was a boy. His only weapon consisted of a stick of mountain mahogeny, about 7 feet long, which had a large knob on one end and a sharpened point at the other. He placed the child in a tree for safety. As the enraged bear made a dash at the Indian, he, jumping skillfully to one side, hit the animal a terrible blow on the legs as it passed. Again and again, as the bear dashed forward, it was struck on the legs until it was nearly disabled, when it was speedily dispatched with the sharp end of the club.

☙ PUFFBALLS

To stop bleeding, the Blackfoot Indians applied the center of dried, unripe puffballs or the powdery center of mature specimens of the same fungus. The Kiowas, a Plains tribe, also used the spores to arrest bleeding from cuts and wounds.

☙ SKUNK CABBAGE

The Menominee Indians prepared a tea by boiling skunk cabbage root hairs and applying it to stop external bleeding. The leaf bases were applied in a wet dressing for bruises by the Meskwakis.

☙ SPIKENARD

The spikenard, a member of the ginseng family, continually reappears in the literature as a favored wound remedy of the native American. The Micmacs, native to New Brunswick and Nova Scotia, and one of the earliest societies of North America contacted by Europeans, prepared a salve of the berries which they used for treating cuts and wounds. The Ojibwas pounded spikenard roots and mixed them with wild ginger as a poultice for treating bone fractures. The Menominees used a poultice of the pounded roots for wounds, while the Potawatomi tribe employed an identical preparation to relieve inflamed areas.

☙ YARROW (FIG.105)

The Ute tribe (after whom the state of Utah is named) held the reputation along with the

(FIG. 105) YARROW: *Ute warriors crushed this common weed between stones and applied it to minor wounds. During the Civil War it became known as soldier's woundwort because of its frequent application to battle wounds.*

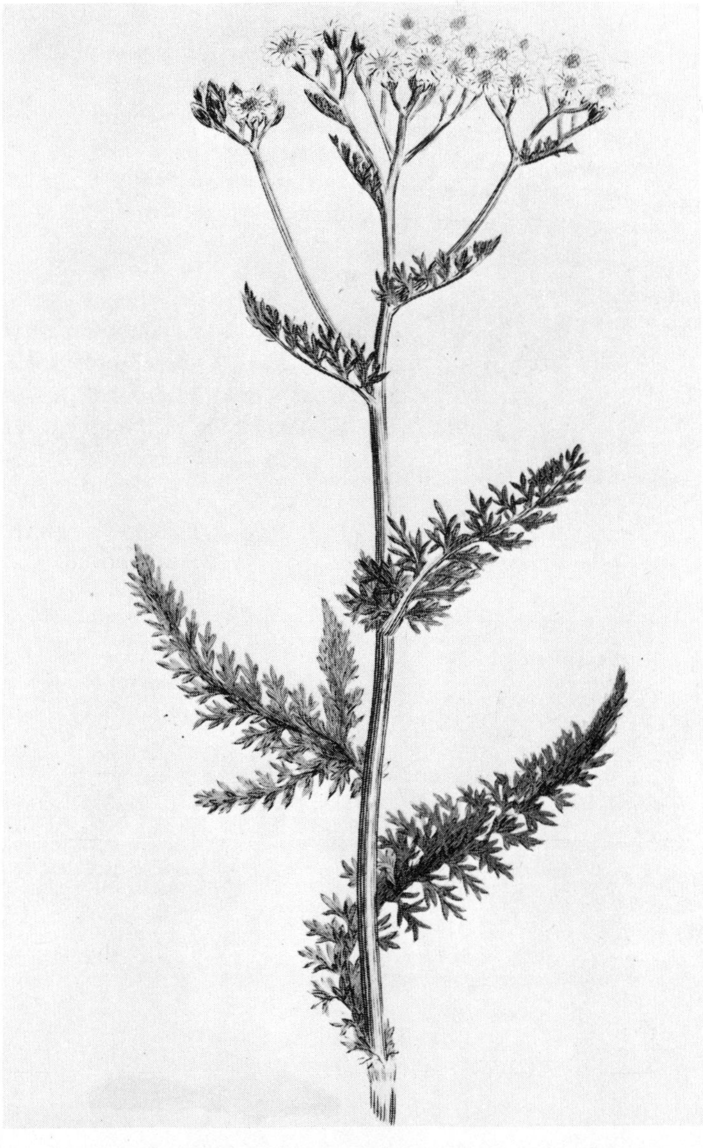

Shoshoni as being the best warriors of the plateau-dwelling Indians. The Ute name for yarrow is translated as "wound medicine"; after pulverizing the yarrow plant, they applied it to cuts, bruises, and other minor injuries. This herb was also used on cuts by the Micmac and Illinois tribes, while the Winnebagos steeped the plant in hot water and used the wash to bathe bruises. The Thompson Indians of British Columbia prepared a powder for dusting on skin sores by roasting the leaves or stems until they were dry enough to be pulverized between stones.

Yarrow is native to the United States and Europe. Its generic name, *Achillea*, is derived from the name of the Greek warrior Achilles. During the Trojan War, an ointment derived from a relative of this plant is said to have been employed to heal the wounds of Achilles' warriors. At one time this species was popularly known as soldier's woundwort by virtue of its value in domestic medicine for treating wounds.

This plant may be found in abandoned fields, along roadsides, and in waste places throughout North America. It grows between one and two feet high, has oblong to lancelike leaves that are divided into numerous slender segments, and numerous small white, pink, or purple flowers which are arranged in a dense, flat-topped cluster. Yarrow may be found in bloom from May to October.

Other plants used in treating wounds include the white pine. The Menominees applied the pounded inner bark as a poultice to cuts, sores, and wounds. The Sioux arrested bleeding with an application of pulverized dried rhizomes of the yellow pond lily, while the Blackfoot Indians used the dried, powdered root of false Solomon's-seal or the crushed leaves of white and purple prairie clover.

Finally, the Zuñi treatment for bullet and arrow wounds, as described by Matilda Stevenson, is included here as an example of the Indian's methods in this area of treatment. The plant employed in this case is *Aster hesperius*, a member of the thistle family, but any of the other plants listed in this section were probably employed in a similar manner by other tribes.

This plant is used also by the Priesthood of the Bow for the treatment of bullet or arrow wounds. A tea is made by boiling the entire plant. If practicable, the missile is removed by squeezing. The wound is washed out with a bit of twisted cloth dipped into the warm tea. When possible the cloth is passed through the cavity of the wound; a slender twig wrapped with raw cotton is then dipped into the tea and the wound is again washed until thoroughly cleansed. Piñon gum, softened by chewing, is made into a pencil, rolled in the powdered root, and inserted into the wound. After withdrawing the gum pencil a quantity of the root powder is sprinkled into the wound; then a pinch of finely ground piñon moistened with spittle is put on the wound, and bandaged in place. This treatment is repeated in the morning and at sunset. Previous to the dressing of the wound each time, if the missile has not been removed the medicine-man endeavors to extract it by pressure. The younger-brother Bow Priest informed the writer that usually not more than two days were required for the extraction of the bullet or arrow by means of this process; but should it not be removed in this way, resort was had to the knife.

MISCELLANEOUS MEDICINES
(Other Indian remedies once official drugs)

ᴇᴊ BLACK ALDER

A fall in the woods requires a quick remedy, to both arrest bleeding and promote healing. Alder bark was used for this purpose by several tribes. The injured party chewed the bark and applied it directly to fresh cuts or bruises. Burns were also soothed by alder, as were inflammations, treated with a bark decoction.

Alders are tannin rich and found in other rational applications. Hemmorhoids and vaginitis were treated with a bark tea, the former ailment receiving the healing liquid via a syringe made of a hollow bone. Dysentery, especially in children, was treated by the Meskwakis by employing a bark decoction. The astringent solution was taken by Menominees suffering from colds, or applied directly on sores.

Herpes infections were successfully treated with bark decoctions or infusions, taken internally and externally, according to a nineteenth-century physician.

ᴇᴊ BLAZING STAR

This interesting indigenous plant, steeped in mystery, was also known as "devil's bit," due to its harsh taste. Somewhat a panacea, the dried roots and rhizome eventually entered into the *National Formulary* between 1916 and 1947, where the plant was listed useful as a diuretic and uterine tonic. Borrowing it from the Indians, eighteenth- and nineteenth-century physicians soon put the plant to use for pains, loss of appetite, and depression ("dejection of spirits"). Alice Henkel, a government scientist of the early twentieth century, thought the blazing star a useful "tonic in derangements of women," according to Vogel.

The genesis of this remedy in American medicine began with an eighteenth-century traveler, Carver, who noted the plant was used "for every

disorder that human nature is incident to, but some of the evil spirits envying mankind the possession of so efficacious a medicine, gave the root a bite, which deprived it of a great part of its virtues."

ᴇᴊ BUCKBEAN

Also known as the marsh trefoil, or water shamrock, this member of the gentian family is a native of Europe and North America. Found from Greenland to Alaska and south to Pennsylvania, Minnesota, and California, all parts of the plant are medicinally active but only the leaves were official: in the *National Formulary*, between 1916 and 1926, and in the *U.S. Pharmacopoeia*, between 1820 and 1842.

Recognized for its fever lowering and tonic properties, Menyanthes was also known to exert cathartic effects. The Kwakiutls boiled the stems and roots and took the resultant decoction for "internal disorders," especially "for spitting blood." Unspecified usage by the Menominees is also reported.

When made up into a tonic, in American domestic medicine 1.3 to 2.0 grams of the powdered leaves or root were used; while an infusion was prepared with half an ounce of the plant to one pint of boiling water, one to two fluid ounces being the dose.

ᴇᴊ CORYDALUS

Pillager Ojibwas suffering from congestion inhaled the smoke of golden corydalus (*C. aurea*), derived from the tubers roasted over hot coals. Related species, such as squirrel corn (*Dicentra canadensis*) and Dutchman's breeches (*D. cucularia*) were utilized by physicians up until the late twentieth century for their tonic properties, also being recommended in venereal diseases.

The dried tubers of these two species of *Dicentra* (known still as "corydalus") were official in the *National Formulary*, between 1916 and 1947. The dose was from 0.65 to 2.0 gm.

✑ HARDHACK

Mohegans treated dysentery with a leaf infusion of this species (*Spiraea tomentosa*), while the Flambean Ojibwas utilized a tea of the flowers and leaves to aid partruition and ameliorate the ill effects of pregnancy.

Many species of this genus contain a volatile oil, similar to oil of wintergreen, composed mainly of salicylic aldehyde with small amounts of methyl salicylate, an aspirin relative. Consequently, at least minimally, the genus *Spiraea* has been used where aspirin is used, for a wide range of complaints. The roots, though, are rich in tannic acid, and found acceptance for the treatment of diarrhea, among the white settlers.

When official in the pharmacopoeia, from 1820 to 1882, hardhack root was recommended in doses of from 0.32–1.3 grams of the water extract repeated *pro re nata*.

✑ INDIAN PHYSIC

Also known as American Ipecac, the roots of this herbaceous plant (*Gillenia trifoliata*) provide a mild and efficient emetic, known to many Indian groups and adopted by the colonists.

The Arkansas tribes used it for bowel complaints, while the Delawares made fit use of the purgative properties.

Official in the *U.S. Pharmacopoeia* from 1820 to 1842 on the primary list, and on the secondary list until 1882, *Gillenia* was recommended in doses of from 1.3 to 2.0 grams of the powdered root. To be maximally potent the root must be gathered in September.

✑ MAGNOLIA

The virtues of this remedy are universally extolled, and even praised for their salutary effects in consumption. The bark being put into brandy, or boiled in any other liquor, is said not only to ease pectoral diseases, but likewise to be of some service against all internal pains and fever, and it could stop dysentery. Persons who had caught cold, boiled the branches of the beaver tree in water, and drank it to their great relief. (Peter Kalm, 1770, in Vogel, *American Indian Medicine*)

Being nearly insoluble in cold, and only slightly soluble in hot water, magnolia bark (*magnolia* species) is very soluble in alcohol. This explains the rationale behind a bitter drink composed of cones of the cucumber tree (*M. acuminata*) in whiskey taken as a preventive against malaria by frontiersmen.

As a fever remedy, for rheumatism, to expel worms, for cramps, the magnolias were long used by various Indian groups.

In the *U.S. Pharmacopoeia* from 1820 to 1894, the dried bark of three species of magnolia (*M. virginiana*, *M. acuminata*, and *M. tripetala*) was recommended in doses of from 2.0 to 3.9 grams of the powdered bark, frequently repeated. The bark loses its powers when dried, however, and is entirely useless when stored for too long.

✑ MUSTARD

Here is an herb long utilized in European folk medicine, and later adopted by the native Americans.

Swallowed whole after being mixed in molasses, mustard seeds (*Brassica*) operate as a laxative. As a condiment, mustard stimulates the gastric mucous membrane and the pancreas.

To relieve headache or toothache, the Mohegans tied the leaves of black mustard (*B. nigra*) directly on the skin. To cure head colds, the Meskwakis sniffed ground mustard seeds.

Mustard plasters are still valued as a rubefacient and must be cautiously applied.

✑ SAGE

California sage (various *Salvia* species) was used throughout its range by Indian healers. To prevent drying of the nasal mucosa, the ground seeds were stirred in water, and the resulting mucilage slowly sucked.

Wild sage (*Salvia lyrata*) was employed by the Catawbas, on the east coast. The roots were pounded into a salve and applied to sores.

Salvia officinalis was entered in the *U.S. Pharmacopoeia* from 1842 to 1916, where it was recommended for its tonic, astringent, and aromatic properties, given in dyspepsia.

Part II

EARTH FOOD

INTRODUCTION TO THE REVISED AND EXPANDED EDITION

Food as Medicine

In all cultures close to the earth, food is medicine. Maintaining health requires a respect for the earth, food, and one's body. When one is out of phase with oneself and ill, medicines, usually in the form of herbs, are next tried. The more drastic techniques, such as surgery, are reserved for extremes, especially the crisis situations that go past the food-medicine plane of healing.

But even there, in the extremes of illness, where surgery is practiced by primitive or nonindustrialized peoples, food is very much part of the recovery. How is it that in Western medicine the importance of eating is just now being rediscovered? How can we expect chain-food restaurant managers to understand and feed sick people when these very same restaurant menus have contributed to the ill-health of the hospitalized patients!

Among the Indian peoples, food has long been part of medical treatment. Cherokee patients, for example, followed strict dietary restrictions. While such food taboos do not make rational sense, the mythological element in healing must never be underestimated. The doctrine that "like cures like" seems here to be reversed, where "*avoiding* like cures like." And so, for example, hot food and salt or plant ash (lye) are almost always restricted during illness, especially in cases of bleeding or when there are sharp pains. The Cherokee medicine man's first prescription was to impose a fast on the patient and kinsfolk, all members of the household being specifically instructed to avoid all hot, cooked food as well as peppers. The theory here was probably that since salt smarts in open wounds, and since hot foods are

scalding, these dietary items tend to aggravate pain.

Rheumatic patients were told to abstain from eating rabbit meat or squirrel owing to the hunchback shape of these animals, while diarrhea was accompanied by a taboo against eating fish or chicken, "because the feces of these animals would seem to indicate that they are chronically afflicted with this very disease" (Mooney, p. 65). Juicy fruit and vegetables were likewise restricted for sufferers of watery blisters.

Cherokee doctors, in sympathy for their patients, avoided all food *themselves* until noon on the day of treatment, but fasted until sundown when treating the seriously ill.

Earth Food

Wild plants have been food staples since antiquity in North America. But even before the Spaniards arrived, corn, beans, pumpkins, and cotton were being cultivated by some Indian groups.

Tribes who were never agricultural peoples lived entirely on wild foods, mainly plants, and animals such as ducks, deer, and antelopes, when they could catch them.

With the coming of the Spanish colonizers, all this changed. Many crops were introduced, enforcing a more sedentary existence on the natives. Nevertheless, the food supply was greatly augmented by wheat, oats, barley, chile, onions, chick peas, peas, new varieties of beans, melons, peaches, apricots, cabbage, lettuce, radishes, carrots, cucumbers, and other crops (Castetter, *Uncultivated Native Plants*, p. 8). By comparison the English-speaking colonists "introduced no plants of importance," only mutton and beef, which the Indians of the Southwest bitterly opposed as food, blaming these symbols of domination for most of their new illnesses.

The great number of wild and cultivated food plants available to the original North Americans, over 1100 species (!), are still there, some in your own corner woodlot. As a resource base these foods must not be forgotten. In the event of war or famine, those knowing where to look will find food sufficient for their survival. In terms of numbers of edible plant *genera*, the top ten families are:

Family	Number of Edible Genera	Rank
Composite (daisy)	45	# 1
Lily	31	# 2
Grasses	27	# 3
Legumes	22	# 4
Umbelliferae (carrot)	20	# 5
Rose	18	# 6
Mint	15	# 7
Ericaceae (heath)	14	# 8
Cruciferae (mustard)	13	# 9
Cactus	12	#10

Again, in terms of numbers, this time of edible *species*, the top ten plant families are:

Family	Number of Edible Species	Rank
Rose	102	# 1
Composite (daisy)	92	# 2
Lily	90	# 3
Legumes	69	# 4
Grasses	47	# 5
Umbelliferae (carrot)	42	# 6
Ericaceae (heath)	41	# 7
Cacti	40	# 8
Pines	33	# 9
Chenopodiaceae (goosefoot)	33	# 9
Beech	32	#10

While it is not likely that other than trained botanists will recognize all edible plants, there are simple rules to follow when lost and hungry!

Rules to Follow When Lost and Hungry
1. All inner tree bark is nutritious.
2. Eat *all* fruits except the bitter.
3. Eat the nuts, washing the acorns repeatedly to remove the tannins.
4. Gather and eat the seeds of grasses.
5. Peas, beans, and lentils are rich in proteins.
6. Salad plants and potherbs: eat them, avoiding the poisonous parsley species. Cook briefly, with little water, changing the water once or twice.
7. Many roots and tubers require boiling (change the water frequently) and sun-drying, and may then be ground into meal.
8. Wild mints and other aromatics make good teas and also add spice.

The Diet of Primitive Man

Many plant foods were and are available, but just *what* primitive man ate must be explored. Can we live only on plant foods; were our ancient ancestors healthier than us; were the Indian peoples paragons of health before being degenerated by the colonizing Europeans? Such questions are important in a book which tends to romanticize "primitive" ways. Owing to the confusion in today's literature about nutrition, an investigation of primitive diet is required.

Surely the pre-Columbian Americans were giants of strength and endurance by contemporary standards, and were rarely plagued by degenerative diseases such as diabetes, heart disease, and so on. Attempting to arrive at a reasonable picture of preindustrial diet and health requires a look at the global evidence. By analyzing primitive diets and disease in antiquity, we will come to see that the plant foods described in this section, while adequate for survival, did by no means constitute the total diet.

Before harking back to a simpler past of evident health perfection, we might evaluate this presumed simplicity of our more natural relatives.

Interesting impressions of prehistoric nutrition come to us from several sources, all within the province of the archaeologist. They are: cave paintings representing plants and animals which we assume were eaten as well as utilized in other ways (as medicines, dyestuffs, fibers, building materials, and so on); the bones of animals, carbonized plant remains, or casts of seeds in clay; the evaluation of gastrointestinal contents of deliberately mummified corpses, or of corpses mummified naturally in extremely dry situations, when frozen or immersed in acid peat bogs; the analysis of coprolites, or prehistoric fecal pellets, usually preserved in dry caves; inferring the food-gathering practices of ancient social groups based on the activities of modern primitive peoples; "chemical archaeology," a method of guessing which plants once grew in archaeological soils by isolating high levels of specific trace elements known to be found in certain species.

Plants as Human Food

Despite these sources of evidence regarding ancient nutrition, the *amount* of information is minimal, which makes generalization difficult. Furthermore, vegetables being perishable, traces of this portion of ancient diets have not been as commonly found as animal remains.

Nevertheless, we do have some knowledge of useful plants in prehistory. Hackberry seeds from Chou-kou-tien in China which are about 500,000 years old are considered the oldest known plant-food remains. Other ancient plant-food finds include unidentified seeds from the site of Terra Amata on the French Riviera, dating some 300,000 years in the past, and several species of seeds and nuts from the site of Kalambo Falls in Africa, dated 100,000 years.

These few archaeological plant samples serve as a partial model for ancient man's plant diet, while the study of coprolites also adds something to our knowledge. Dried fecal pellets analyzed from sites in Israel, Peru, Chile, the western United States, Mexico, Kentucky, and Arkansas suggest the dominant role played by plant food.

Michael Kliks, a Berkeley parasitologist, has studied coprolites from Lovelock Cave, Nevada, and believes that anthelmintic substances found in seeds of the genus *Chenopodium* (wormwood) account for the absence of intestinal worms in these people. His examination also revealed that these coprolites were composed of up to 30 percent fibrous residues, indicating a high vegetable diet.

Another method useful for guessing at ancient diets is pollen analysis of archaeological site soils. But we are doomed to an incomplete guess because we may learn much about the ground vegetation without knowing if any of these plants were actually eaten.

While little is certain concerning the exact value of plant foods in ancient and prehistoric diets, we must assume that the more than 500,000 species of flowering plants provided many nutritious seeds, fruits, leaves, and roots. When we add the "lower" plants (algae, fungi, conifers, and such), respectable vegetarian regimens can be constructed for most of man's known geographical niches.

Animals as Human Food

It is much easier to prove that meat and other animal foods, rather than plants, played a major role in prehistoric nutrition. Stone tools presumably used for killing prey, and the bones of creatures consumed, come to us in good states of preservation. There is documentation of meat eating from Olduvai Gorge in Bed 1, dating approximately 1.8 million years. In some Olduvai localities the bones of one species are found; in others, the bones of several animal species are witness to early dietary histories.

The justification for examining nutrition in contemporary primitive groups is that they may be more similar to ancient peoples than are contemporary "civilized" men. From the practices of some contemporary primitive peoples we know *how much* meat can be eaten by hungry hunters. An anthropologist in Brazil watched four Siriono men eat a sixty-pound peccary at one time! Holmberg estimated that each party ate about ten pounds of food, while in another situation he saw two men eat six spider monkeys in a single day. Each monkey weighed ten to fifteen pounds, so his estimate of thirty pounds (!) of meat in twenty-four hours per man seems plausible. In the 1930s, Stefansson reported that Point Barrow Eskimos ate about nine pounds of uncooked seal meat on a daily basis (with little vegetable food in their overall diet; the vitamin C is gained from the animal's intestinal flora, algae, and other seal-eaten vegetables).

Vogel reports that Loskiel, a writer who visited North America in the late eighteenth century, wrote, "An Indian makes nothing of dragging a deer of one hundred or one hundred and fifty pounds weight home, through a very considerable tract of forest."

Man as Human Food

Cannibalism is sometimes offered as "proof" that man has high protein requirements which, when frustrated, force him to consume his own kind, even portions of his own body. Yet the purely ritualistic elements of this practice must not be underplayed. *Sinanthropus*, who dates 500,000 years back, is the first group known to have cannibalized, or at least sacrificed, his neighbor. It is fairly well established that the Aztecs sacrificed and ate more than 500,000 people each year, perhaps to increase the supply of animal protein in a region denuded of wild game, to reduce population pressures, or simply to release violent energies in an otherwise civil society. Cannibalism still prevails in remote New Guinea valleys, and until this century cases of cannibalism were reported in peaceful Fiji. Whether humans, or "long pig," were eaten for nutritional values, to express victorious sentiments, or to contain population growth, are questions which must remain buried and unanswered in the earth's crust.

Is Man an Omnivore?

In attempting to establish a rational diet for contemporary man, arguments are posed on both sides of the animal-vegetable question. One group holds that we as a species are basically meat eaters, another finds the herbivore model appealing, while our anatomy, notably our small canines and long digestive tract, suggest we were made for a vegetable diet which requires lengthy digestion.

The Old Testament, which was apparently written about 5,700 years ago, is an excellent ethnological document. By this time we see man's omnivorous balance clearly recorded.

Insects as Human Food

We know from contemporary tribal peoples just how valuable edible insects are nutritionally. The Pedi people eat many insect species, about which a great deal is known. This information indicates that ancient peoples likely ate insects whenever they could be gotten.

As an example of the food value of the insects, the nutritional composition of fresh, whole caterpillars is average unit weight, 10.2 grams; mois-

ture, 85.0 percent; protein, 8.3 percent (Quin, 1959).

The Pedi eat live caterpillars, pupa, and larva, generally after roasting them in live cinders for about fifteen minutes. These caterpillars are so popular that they are bought by native traders for retailing in other areas. Other insects eaten on a regular basis include beetles (30.3 percent protein), grasshoppers (29.2 percent protein), locusts (18.2 percent protein; legs alone: 55.5 percent protein), and ants (males 25.2 percent; females 7.4 percent protein). Elsewhere, insects eaten in primitive diets include waterbugs and caterpillars. The last-named insects are excellent sources of nutrients and play a significant role in the diet of many peoples, including the Bemba of northern Rhodesia. (The famous eighteenth-century astronomer, De Lalande, frequented the naturalist Quatremere D'Isjonvalle, "to feast on caterpillars which he claimed tasted like stone-fruits.")

Many other insects and insect relatives are consumed by the Pedi, including the praying mantis, scorpions, spiders, and termites, a universal primitive food. Insects considered repugnant and *not* eaten by the Pedi include lice and cockroaches. But in Thailand two roach species and their eggs are eaten, while the Chinese are said to have relied upon this pest as well. The topic of *Insects as Human Food* is well treated by Bodenheimer, who adds an interesting anecdote about the larvae of a *Hepialid* moth eaten by the Mundracos of Central America for the acute intoxication which results. The point is, insects have figured prominently as human food. They are excellent protein sources, and only Western cultural conditioning limits their wider utilization as human food.

And the fear of you and the dread of you shall be upon every beast of the earth, and upon every fowl of the air, and upon all wherewith the ground teemeth, and upon all the fishes of the sea: into your hand are they delivered. Every moving thing that liveth shall be for food for you; as the green herb have I given you all. Only flesh with the life thereof, which is the blood thereof, shall ye not eat. (*Genesis* 9:2–4)

Tools and Diet

Our progressive development of tools and techniques gradually altered the type of foods eaten, providing a greater variety and probably a more certain supply. In "Man, the Hunter-Gatherer," Heizer states that "the earliest pebble tools, dating from about 2,000,000 years ago, provided 5 cm of cutting edge per pound of flint. In the Lower Paleolithic (500,000 to 1,000,000 years ago), the implement cutting edge per pound of raw material rises to 20 cm; in the Middle Paleolithic, the figure is 100 cm; and in the Upper Paleolithic, it reached 300 to 1200 cm." This progression in efficiency of tool production must have yielded more and better prepared food, somewhat akin to more efficient automobiles which give us more miles per gallon and, hopefully, better ride.

Heizer wisely argues that "while there are some examples of tool use among lower animals—the Galapagos finch, for example, which uses a cactus thorn held in its beak to spear grubs and extract them from their holes; or the African vulture, which uses a stone, again held in the beak, to hammer open ostrich eggs; or the sea otter, which uses pebbles to break apart mollusk shells—none of these animals actually forms or fashions implements from wood or stone to serve a specific purpose. Only man does this." In so doing, pre-Neolithic and many of the less complex agricultural societies thus earn the title "hunter-gatherer," clearly standing apart from the lower animals.

Yet we must not be too quick to conclude that the development of tools and other technology *necessarily* produced a more desirable nutritional balance. The introduction of subsistence agriculture tends to *reduce* the number of species eaten. Primitive hunting peoples eat from a wide range of animal and plant species, and tend to eat the whole of the edible portion, such as the marrow and organs of animals, the seeds and skins of fruits. Such a diverse diet would be expected to be fairly well balanced because nutrients are unevenly distributed in foods, only many different foods making up a whole.

When populations shift to cash-crop agriculture or wage-earning, and where overly refined foods form a large part of the diet, dangerous deficiency diseases result. Beri-beri in the Far East and kwashiorkor in Africa have increased in prevalence with modernization and technological "improvements." We know that kwashiorkor is uncommon among primitive peoples who normally practice mixed farming but is common in areas where a cash-crop economy is king. Asians who eat little but polished rice suffer much from beri-beri, a disease rare in areas where home-pounded brown rice is the staple.

However, not all contemporary primitives eat well-balanced diets. The Papuan New Guinea highlanders depend on the sweet potato for 90 percent of caloric and 50 percent of protein needs. Some animal protein is eaten, but not enough, for kwashiorkor is endemic. Australian aboriginal people have experienced scurvy epidemics, especially during droughts. Primitive peoples are often hungry, and famine due to warfare, epidemics, or climate is not uncommon. The porotic hyperostosis discovered among the ancient Hopis was likely due to a lack of iron.

Disease in Antiquity

Skeletal remains do not supply the whole picture of ancient diets and health. We know, for example, that custom and belief may lead to the neglect of nutritionally valuable foods. As Barnicot points out, eggs and fish are frequently avoided in contemporary human societies, while "animals, such as pigs in New Guinea and cattle in many African pastoral peoples, are often desired more for prestige than as sources of meat." Further, variations in bone density have not been studied to any extent in excavated skeletal material. Yet, bone density variations that have been recorded in contemporary human populations may be related to diet. A study of the now extinct Sadlermiut Eskimos, revealed that their specialized animal-food diet influenced their high bone densities. Studies on ancient diet and skeletons, then, must at this time "refer to certain well-defined abnormalities detectable in bones or teeth, and to certain historic references to early population health."

In *Diseases in Antiquity*, Brothwell clearly defines well-known dietary deficiencies discovered in skeletal remains in the following categories:

Vitamin D deficiency. Rickets, caused by a lack of this vitamin, produces pronounced skeletal deformities such as bowing of the femur, tibia, and fibula. The examination of many, many prehistoric and protohistoric skeletons from Europe and North Africa shows little evidence of this deficiency disease. Similar investigations among the mummies of twenty-nine children under fourteen years of age from pre-Columbian Peru by Moodie yielded not a trace of the disease. This led him to conclude that since "the disease was not found among the ancient Egyptians . . . , like syphilis, rickets apparently is a modern disease."

Skeletons from London, c. 1750–1850, known as the "St. Brides's Church skeletal series," show rickets deformity in 6.9 percent of 233 remains. Brothwell is not convinced that this proves the disease appeared only after the industrial revolution and cites the facts "that Soranus of Ephesus (A.D. 98–138) refers to rachitic-like deformities of the legs in children in Italy, while Chinese literature of the third century B.C. refers to crooked legs and hunchback." Perhaps these early cereal cultivators who ate high carbohydrate diets were wise enough to include fish, dairy foods, and sunlight in their overall scheme of health.

Vitamin C deficiency. There is not much evidence of deficiency diseases related to this vitamin in skeletal remains, probably owing to the wide omnivorous diet of early hunting-collecting peoples. Early cultivators also probably consumed ample quantities of ascorbic acid from fruit, vegetables, and wild edible leaves used as potherbs.

The Pedi people, a Southern African agricultural people visited by Quin in the 1950s, ate many greens which are known to be good sources of the antiscorbutic vitamin. As an example, the common pigweed (*Amaranthus* sp.) ranges from 0.6 to 3.0 mg ascorbic acid per gram, as compared with 0.4 to 0.6 mg per cc for orange juice or lemon juice. Cultivated plants also provided much vita-

min C, such as the runner tips of the pumpkin plant, which were found to contain 45.6 mg per 100 gm, or tender cow-pea leaves, which yielded 103 mg per 100 g. The Pedi intuitively knew that the young, tender plant parts were better nutritionally than old leaves (probably because they taste better), and selected only young materials for consumption. An average meal was found to contain about 27 mg ascorbic acid, just from greens. Further, to digress a moment, the mineral content of pigweed and other greens is so significant as to contain more calcium than milk!

Thus, even surviving primitive agricultural people consume vitamin C in generous amounts. We would expect that the earliest Americans consumed even *more* of this vitamin via wild greens consumption, not only as food, but through the frequent consumption of herbal medicines, an often overlooked nutritional input. My ethnomedical investigations in Fiji showed a very high incidence of "bush-tea" consumption, for complaints ranging from headache to diabetes. Since most wild herbs are rich in vitamins, including vitamin C, these "teas" would contribute much vitamin nutrition, usually unobserved in standard dietary surveys. This observation tends to support the contention of Linus Pauling, who believes that our distant ancestors consumed enormous amounts of this vitamin, thereby supporting his claim for our megavitamin needs.

Yet we must not rush to conclude that all ancient peoples were fortified with this essential vitamin. Despite the assumed lack of vitamin C-related diseases in prehistory, Brothwell suggests that "the relatively numerous cases of vertebral

Mineral Content of Common Plants
Grams per 100 g (3 oz) of Foodstuff

	Water	Mineral Salts	Calcium	Magnesium	Iron
Milk	87.0	0.7	0.12	0.012	0.00024
Cabbage	91.5	1.0	0.045	0.015	0.001
Lettuce	94.7	0.9	0.043	0.017	0.0007
Lucerne	82.0	1.6	0.36	0.07	0.008
Spinach	92.0	2.1	0.07	0.04	0.004
Black Jack	80.0	2.2	0.61	0.18	0.01
Pigweed	75.0	4.1	0.65	0.52	0.02

(Quin, 1959)

collapse in Amerindian skeletons might have resulted from scurvy. . . . They are not all the result of senile osteoporosis."

Vitamin A and B-complex deficiencies. The bones are unaffected by deficiencies of these vitamins, but there are early records of disorders related to such deficiencies. Night blindness, or nyctalopia, is mentioned in the *Ebers Papyrus* (c. 1600 B.C.), by Hippocrates, and later in Chinese medical books (A.D. 610). Cereal cultivators with little animal protein would be especially vulnerable to this disorder. The symptoms of vitamin B-1 deficiency—beri-beri—are outlined in the *Su Wen*, a Chinese treatise of c. 2690 B.C. During the extended siege of T'ai Ch'eng (A.D. 529) over 100,000 of a total population of 120,000 people manifested symptoms of the disease—swelling of the body, difficulty breathing—and died. This shows how extensive the disease can become with deficient diets. The same condition is mentioned by Strabo in his commentary on Roman troops.

Iodine insufficiency. Thyroid malfunction in regions with iodine deficient soils would have resulted in cretinism. We do not have direct skeletal evidence of this disorder, but many sedentary peoples of the post-mesolithic period could have possibly suffered from a lack of iodine. Endemic goiter in remote Alpine regions was recorded by Pliny, an indication of the possibility of widespread manifestation of the disorder during more ancient times.

Overspecializing and disease. The effects of famine on human health needs no elucidation. The Chinese people, for example, suffered over 1800 famines for the period 100 B.C. to A.D. 1910. During famines, people ingeniously adapt themselves to little-favored foods. First-century-B.C. Chinese grew the water darnel, a drought and flood resistant weed, to carry them through lean times.

Analyzing the effects of deficiency diseases and famine does not tell the whole story. We must also see how relying too strongly on one particular food can result in nutrient deficiencies. For example, the pulse *Lathyrus sativus*, a drought resistant pea, has been eaten excessively during famines in regions of Africa, Asia, and southern Europe. A toxic constituent of this food can bring about paralysis of the legs, as recorded by Hippocrates: "At Ainos, all men and women who con-tinuously ate peas, became impotent in the legs and in that state perished."

Similarly, the excessive utilization of fava beans (*Vicia faba*) produces favism, a blood condition. Also known as broad beans or horse beans, they were grown and eaten in ancient Egypt, having been uncovered in the tombs of the pharaohs from the Fifth and Sixth Dynasties, circa 2,000 B.C. Surprisingly, ancient Greek athletes were encouraged to eat this food to improve their athletic prowess.

Fava bean hemolysis does not occur in every individual who eats this food. Genetic factors in man play a role, as do the effects of cooking, digestion, absorption, and elimination. As with many toxic foods, the susceptibility to and severity of the toxic effects vary from individual to individual. There are no absolutes, even with hemolytic plant poisons.

Overemphasizing the values of any one food can produce problems, even in a substance generally recognized as safe, such as honey. There have been reports since antiquity of poisonings from eating certain honeys. Plants which produce toxic honey include the mountain laurel, azalea, and species of rhododendron. In the nineteenth century, a cluster of deaths occurred in Branchville, South Carolina, as a result of eating yellow jasmine honey.

Dental health and diet. Caries has been seen in skeletal remains of fossil man. Neolithic dental remains show no real increase in caries rate above those of paleolithic and mesolithic populations, despite the advent of agriculture.

Iron Age people show an increased caries rate, while the British Bronze Age apparently shows a lower rate than the neolithic. This leads one archaeologist to speculate that the earlier people relied less on grains than the latter group. Grain-eating people generally show greater tooth loss, more caries, and less tooth wear than hunting-collecting groups. Unbalanced or inadequate diets may influence periodontal disease in other ways, by increased calculus deposits and tooth abrasion resulting from a high carbohydrate diet, and by bringing about protein deficiency periodontitis. A study of early Egyptian skeletons shows an increase of alveolar bone loss, a clear mark of periodontal disease, from predynastic to late dynastic times. This was no doubt related to diet.

As populations shifted from hunting and leaf-berry eating and increased their consumption of cereals, teeth decayed more often and tooth enamel diminished. Whether this resulted from the high-grain diet per se, or from a lack of vitamins, minerals, and protein, remains to be determined. The point is, an increasing dependence on carbohydrates, be they from cultivated grains or from naturally occurring sources, generally correlates with decreased dental health. A study of many prehistoric central California Indian skeletons, from individuals who lived between 2000 B.C. and A.D. 1500, shows an increase in dental caries. This correlates with a shift in dependence on collecting and hunting and an increasing reliance on the acorn.

Other diseases in antiquity. In constructing our model of ancient health, it is always tempting to take extreme positions, firm evidence not being abundant. One school generally holds that our earliest relatives were all healthy animals and that only with industrialization have most of our grave degenerative diseases originated. Another school, the optimists, likes to believe that mankind has enjoyed an increasing degree of health and longevity as a result of "progress" and modern sanitation.

Statistics do not lie; man does.

Judging from skeletal remains, mean life expectancy for neolithic adults was about twenty-eight to thirty-one years for females and about thirty-one to thirty-four years for males. About a century ago, a significant *increase* of life expectancy occurred, mainly in the industrialized world. How do we interpret these figures? Can we say with any certainty that our neolithic life-expectancy figures are truly representative? We must remember how high infant-mortality rates are in contemporary primitive societies, and also how many neolithics represented by the skeletons used to compute the above life expectancies died *not* from nutrition-related diseases, but from accident and injury.

In either case, it is important to remember that many of mankind's most horrible ills have been with the species since antiquity, and cannot therefore be the product of industrialization. Polishing grains and robbing them of their B vitamins may not add to our health (!), but we cannot say that like processes are the *cause* of most of our ills.

Neoplasms *did* exist in antiquity, as skeletal evidence well demonstrates. Primary benign tumors are evidenced in the remains of many ancient dead, including ivory osteomata (small circular mounds) in Egyptians of Roman date, and in early Pecos Pueblo Indians. Malignant tumors of bone are to be found in a Lower/Middle Pleistocene skull; a pelvic tumor is seen in the remains from the catacombs of Kom el-Shougafa in Alexandria; osteogenic sarcoma is described in an Iron Age skeleton from Munsingen, Switzerland; and so on with other examples from antiquity.

Primary carcinomas and secondary involvement of bones have been tentatively identified from the Iranian site of Tepe Hissar, where a portion of a destroyed jaw (3500–3000 B.C.) was found. A large frontal tumor centered over the left orbit has been noted in a pre-Hispanic Peruvian skull, while literature tells us that Domecedes of Crotona (520 B.C.) healed a woman of breast cancer.

Renal calculi, or kidney stones, were found in a predynastic Egyptian mummy. Analysis showed they were composed of mixed phosphates and uric acid and that they were probably in the bladder.

There is also some evidence that endocrine diseases, diabetes mellitus, goiter, and exophthalmos existed in antiquity. Barrenness was definitely a problem, spontaneous abortion occurred, and many "gynecological complaints—amenorrhea, leucorrhea, menorrhagia, prolapse of the uterus, diseases of the cervix, of the body of the uterus, and of the vulva—were probably as frequent as they are in present-day practice." Also, male urethritis was fairly common among the ancients.

We can go on with a long list of diseases prevalent in ancient societies, the point being that our medical problems were not born with a shift from the wilderness to civilization and its many discontents. Certainly, many modern food-processing techniques do not add to our nutrient level; sugar, fats, salt and chemical additives are *not* desirable in our foods. But we must not rush to judgment following the Pied Pipers of health faddism, who would have us believe we would all live to the age of Moses should we follow their brand of Messianic nutrition.

And so, having examined the archaeological record and early literature, we see that prehistoric and later records of human nutrition invite some strong conclusions. Man the hunting-collecting food gatherer existed largely on fruit and vegetables with *occasional* high-protein feasts of animal protein. It is foolish to argue that early man subsisted on meat; as any hunter will tell you, the catch is not always assured. A day-to-day diet of *leaves* would have been the only sure thing, except in polar regions. Anatomically we have a mid-length gut and small canines, indicating an omnivorous diet as desirable. Human diets vary immensely, and the things which are regarded as fit to eat also vary greatly from culture to culture.

The rich botanical base of North America was a bounty of food for our Indian predecessors and remains so for those of us who seek foods of the earth.

THE ACORNS AND OTHER NUTS
(Beech, Walnut, and Soapberry Families)

❧ BEECH

Beechnuts, which are up to 22 percent protein, were an important part of the Iroquois diet. The sweet and edible kernels were either eaten fresh, after having been prepared the same way as that described below for acorns, or they were stored for times of scarcity. Usage is reported among tribes of the eastern and north central states. The Indians of Maine even utilized the immature nut for food.

The Latin name for the beeches, *Fagus*, comes from the Greek word meaning "to eat." It is conjectured that beechnuts were once a primary food of mankind.

Although not employed by the Indians as a substitute for coffee, roasted beechnuts were adapted for this purpose by the early settlers. The inner bark of the beech tree has been used, like pine, to make bread.

❧ CHESTNUT

The Iroquois gathered fresh chestnuts, removed the outer shells, and then crushed the kernels in wooden bowls. The crushed nuts were then boiled in water and the oil skimmed off the surface. This delicious oil was served separately with corn bread and used as a topping for various puddings. The remaining boiled nutmeat was used to make puddings, or when dried, was pounded into flour and added to bread ingredients to produce a better flavor.

The chestnut kernel is approximately 7 percent fat and 11 percent protein and contains phosphorus, potassium, magnesium, and sulphur.

A close relative of the American chestnut, the chinquapin, produces a smaller, sweeter nut, which was eaten by Indian groups throughout its range of growth, from Texas to Pennsylvania.

The American chestnut originally extended throughout New England, north to Ontario, but was destroyed by a chestnut blight. The great forests of American chestnuts have been replaced by new plantings of Asian varieties. The common chestnuts sold by street vendors in many American cities are mainly imported from Spain and Italy.

❧ OAK (FIG.106)

The acorns were the most important nut food of most Indian tribes. To render the tender nutmeat palatable, it is first necessary to remove the bitter and constipating tannin. V. K. Chestnut visited the Indians of Mendocino County, California, in the late 1890s and recorded their method for removing this bitter principle. He also described their method for converting acorn kernels into flour. Since these methods employed by the Indians of northern California were similar to those of most tribes of North America, they are worth including nearly in their entirety.

The broad and stately White Oak is the most characteristic tree of the best farming land of the region, but in every locality throughout the county there are one or more different species of oak which furnish in good seasons a great abundance of acorns, which although not edible in the raw condition, are converted by simple processes into a very satisfying and wholesome diet. The Concows especially, who are not used to eating much meat, claim that they never get sick from eating the mush and bread made from acorns. As a class these nuts are oily, and hence they replace in a measure the oily fish more largely consumed by the coast Indians.

One simple method for removing the tannin was "occasionally accomplished by burying the acorns in a sandy place with grass, charcoal, and ashes, and then soaking them in water from time to time until they become sweet."

To make soup and bread the Indians of Round

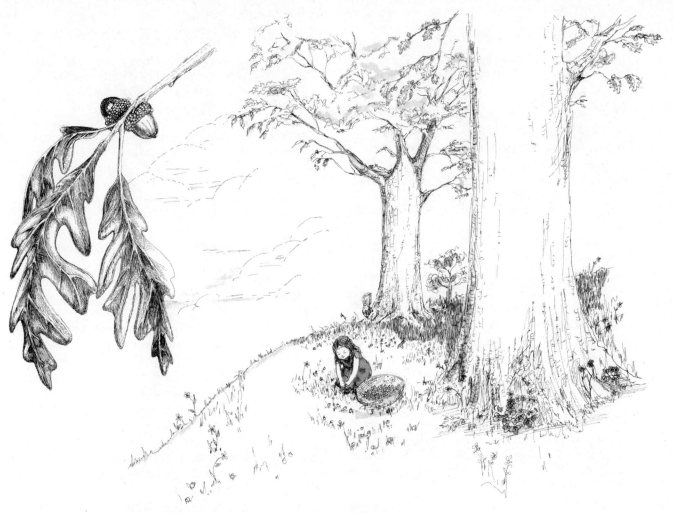

(FIG. 106) WHITE OAK: *Mush and bread made from acorns was an important Indian food. To remove the bitter tannin, several methods of leaching were practiced.*

Valley first dried the nuts in the sun and then, through considerable effort, rendered them into a fine meal by use of a stone mortar.

Mr. Chestnut continues by describing how the bitter tannin was removed:

[The meal was mixed] with water in a shallow depression which is made in sand or some porous material and . . . the water [was allowed] to percolate through the mass until the bitter taste has disappeared. A couple of hours are usually required for the operation . . . The acorn meal after this process has the consistency of ordinary dough. It is sometimes converted into bread while still in the sand by building a fire around it; but this method is objectionable on account of the sand which adheres to the bread and the loss of the oil . . . A considerable quantity is scooped out from the center of the depression; and this, which is entirely free from sand, is reserved and

afterwards made into bread. The remainder of the dough . . . is rubbed up with . . . water . . . and this is converted into soup.

The dough selected for acorn bread is mixed with red clay before it is baked, the proportion being about 1 pound of clay to 20 of dough. This clay, several Indians explained, makes the bread sweet. Others stated that it "acted like yeast." The mixture is placed on a bed of Soaproot, Oak, Maple, or even Poison-Oak leaves, which in turn rests on a bed of rocks previously heated by a small fire. The dough is then covered with leaves and a layer of hot rocks and dirt and cooked gently in this primitive oven for about twelve hours, usually over night. When removed the next morning the bread, if previously mixed with clay, is as black as jet, and, while still fresh, has the consistency of rather soft cheese. In the course of a few days it becomes hard, when, on account of the leaf impressions stamped upon it, it might easily be mistaken for a fossil-bearing piece of coal.

We learn from H. H. Smith, the ethnobotanist, that John Muir, the great naturalist, "during his arduous tramps in the mountains of California, often carried the hard, dry acorn bread of the Indians and deemed it the most compact and strength-giving food he had ever used."

Smith relates that "The Acorns were . . . so important that Oaks which produced abundant crops were considered, among most of the Pomo Indians of California, to be personal property. The ownership of these trees was passed down in the family in accordance with definite rules."

In Wisconsin, the Menominee Indians used roasted and ground acorns of the northern pin oak as a coffee substitute.

Acorn meal of white oak is about 6 percent protein and 65 percent total carbohydrates.

This nourishing food has been used since early times in Greece and France. It appears as if the Europeans were aware of the value of these nuts. As Fernald and Kinsey write, these are the words of an English writer: "And Men had indeed *Hearts of Oak*; I mean, not so *hard*, but *health*, and *strength*, and liv'd naturally, and with things easily *parable* and plain."

The bitternut, butternut, hickory, pecan, pignut, and walnut all belong to the walnut family. All were used to some extent by the Indians, but the Iroquois use is the most interesting variation on the theme of native nut foods.

A. C. Parker, the anthropologist of Seneca Iroquois ancestry, relates how his people cracked tough shells by placing the nuts in depressions that had been cut into boulders or shale specifically for this purpose and then hitting them with a solid stone.

The Senecas made a baby food by mixing the dried, pulverized kernels of butternut and hickory with dried, pulverized deer or bear meat. This dried mixture was added to boiling water and then fed to hungry infants.

The nursing bottle was a dried and greased beargut. The nipple was a bird's quill around which was tied the gut to give proper size. To clean these bottles they were untied at both ends, turned wrong side out, rinsed in warm water, thrown into cold water, shaken and hung in the smoke to dry.

Another nut-bearing tree, the shrubby California buckeye, or horse chestnut, was practically a food staple among the Indians of California. This tree belongs to another family entirely, but bears large nuts which are edible after considerable preparation.

The starchy raw nuts contain the bitter principle aesculin, which has had some use as a fish stupefier. One California tribe ate these nuts to commit suicide. To remove this poison from the nut, several variations on the theme of roasting and leaching were followed. The nuts were first placed in a pit lined with hot stones and covered with willow leaves and hot ashes, and baked from one to ten hours. They were then removed, shelled, sliced into thin pieces, and placed in a container in a stream for two to five days. A shorter leaching process was effected by mashing the roasted nuts with water and then soaking them for only one to ten hours in a sand pit along the bank of a stream. The pulpy mass was then eaten without further preparation. The buckeyes were not preserved for winter use because they sprout very quickly and lose their agreeable taste.

Although several species of buckeye grow in the eastern United States, the California variety produced the nut most frequently eaten by the Indians. It is a broad, spreading tree that grows between ten and forty feet in height. From May to July, it bears numerous clusters of fragrant white blossoms that are followed, in the fall, by the large nutritious nuts. These are about 23 percent protein and are worth preparing, especially in situations where animal protein is unavailable or not desired.

THE BEANS AND PEAS

The immense group of bean plants provided the Indian with foods that were highly regarded, the beans being second in importance only to corn. Many bean plants have been cultivated in America since pre-Columbian times, some tribes growing more than ten varieties which they claimed were of ancient origin.

In the East, the bush bean, the kidney bean, and varieties of the wild pea served as food, while in the West, and especially in the arid regions of New Mexico, Texas, Arizona, Utah, Nevada, and California, a most valuable survival food, the mesquite, provided a "flour" that has been considered by at least one writer to be "the most nutritious breadstuff in use among any people."

The bean family includes widely diverse species of vines, trees, shrubs, and herbs that grow in diverse environments, ranging from wet forests to deserts. Many of these plants are able to survive in poor soil, and when they decay, they contribute great quantities of nitrogen to the soil.

In addition to providing the native American with important foods in the form of seeds, pods, and legumes, some of these plants provided him with drugs, insecticides, tools, timber for construction, firewood, and fodder for his animals.

ALFALFA

Indians of Utah ground alfalfa seeds between stones and cooked this "flour" as mush or bread. They also boiled new branches and ate them as greens.

Alfalfa leaf is very rich in vitamin K; it has been used in medicine to encourage the clotting of blood. This has been especially valuable as a "natural" cure for jaundice.

Alfalfa leaf is also an excellent source of vitamins A and D and is used in Pablum, a popular infants' cereal.

The leaves are best collected in the spring or early summer and eaten fresh, in salads, or steeped in hot water and drunk as a tea.

BEACH PEA

The Iroquois ate the sprouts and stalks of young beach pea plants, which were less than ten inches high, as greens. This plant contains seeds which resemble green peas. Although the ripe peas have been eaten in emergencies, some people say they are slightly poisonous. In any case the shoots commonly grow in the sand of beaches in the eastern United States and are edible after boiling. It is possible that the Iroquois were aware of the poisonous nature of certain varieties of this pea and selected only the young, small plants because they lacked the poisonous principle.

Other varieties of the wild pea were eaten by tribes across the states. In California, a scrambling vine variety with yellowish brown flowers was eaten by the Yokia Indians. However, again, only the small plants, about three inches high, were chosen and cooked for greens. At the turn of the century this plant was described as growing so intensely in Round Valley that it made walking difficult.

INDIAN BREADROOT (FIG. 107)

The large, white, starchy Indian breadroot roots were prepared by the Indians of the West in various ways. The plants were gathered in midsummer when the leaves were dry and beginning to turn brown, and the roots were eaten raw, peeled and roasted, or boiled. Occasionally, they were dried and ground into a flour, which was baked into cakes or used for gruel or as a seasoning.

The breadroot was one of the most important economic plants of the Plains tribes. There, it grew on the dry prairie in hard soil and was very difficult to gather. The plant parts which appear above ground level were blown away by the strong winds soon after they ripened. This made it important to gather the roots while the plant was still visible.

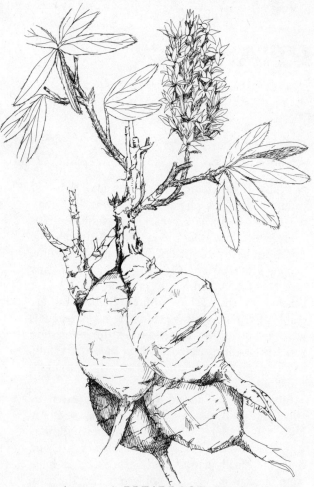

(FIG. 107) BREADROOT: *The large, white, starchy root was eaten raw, roasted, or boiled. These roots so impressed an early French explorer that he attempted to establish this plant as an important food crop in Europe.*

An early French explorer was so impressed by these white, starchy roots that he sent the plant back to France, around 1800, in the hope of establishing it as an important food crop. Breadroot was not well received, and the industry failed to materialize; nevertheless, this root has saved many men in America from starvation, and is still valued as an excellent survival food.

❧ CLOVER

Clover has been used extensively as fodder and was eaten by the Indians in several ways. The foliage was eaten fresh, before flowering, and was generally picked from April through July by the Indians of northern California, who valued it highly. The Digger tribe cooked red clover by placing several moistened layers upon one an-

other in a stone oven. The Apaches boiled clover together with dandelions, grass, and pigweed.

Clover appears to have been important to the native Americans, for as Sturtevant shows: "Where clover is found growing wild, the Indians practice a sort of semicultivation by irrigating it and harvesting."

The leaves contain many of the essential food ingredients; however, they have been known to cause bloating in human beings as well as in cattle. Chestnut stated that the Indians ate pepper nuts or dipped clover in salt water to aid its digestion and to prevent the bloating.

The Pomo tribe held special clover feasts and dances in the early spring to celebrate the appearance of this food plant. As Barrett related: "The people moved out into the fields and reveled in the abundance of these greens, eating great quantities as they gathered them, and bringing them back to the village by the basketful."

The use of clover as human food was not limited to the North American Indian. In Ireland and Scotland the dried flowers and seeds of the common white clover were ground into a nutritious bread.

A recent medical report from the Mayo Clinic, as contained in Harris's book, indicates that sweet clover contains an effective anticoagulent that may find application in treating coronary thrombosis.

❧ GROUNDNUT (INDIAN POTATO)

The groundnut vine is found throughout New England and extends south to Florida and Texas and west to Montana. The Indians showed this plant to the Pilgrims, and during their first winter in New England, these Europeans subsisted entirely on the tubers, either raw or boiled.

The value of this plant spread quickly among the arriving settlers, and as early as 1635, it was brought to Europe and cultivated in France.

As is typical, after the Indians saved the lives of the Pilgrims by showing them how to survive on the groundnut, by 1654 a law was passed which forbade the Indian from digging these tubers on "English land." For a first offense the native American was liable to be jailed, and for a second, whipping was the reward.

An early visitor to North America, Peter Kalm, wrote about this tuberous plant in his journal:

Hopniss, or *Hapniss*, was the Indian name of a wild plant which they ate . . . The Swedes in New Jersey and Pennsylvania still call it by that name, and it grows in the meadows in a good soil. The roots resemble potatoes, and were boiled by the Indians . . . Mr. Bartram told me that the Indians who live farther in the country do not only eat these roots, which are equal in goodness to potatoes, but likewise take the peas which lie in the pods of this plant and prepare them like common peas.

The groundnut was extremely important so far as nutritive value is concerned, providing up to 18 percent protein by weight.

◡§ HOG PEANUT (FIG. 108)

The underground fruits of the twining hog peanut vine were eaten in large quantities by Indians of the eastern and central United States. The tough outer shell is easily removed by boiling when the nutritious beans are exposed. Hog peanuts are approximately 25 percent protein, the highest protein yield of any wild plant consumed by the Indians.

(FIG. 108) *HOG PEANUT: These underground fruits contain about 25 percent protein, the highest amount found in any wild plant consumed by the Indians.*

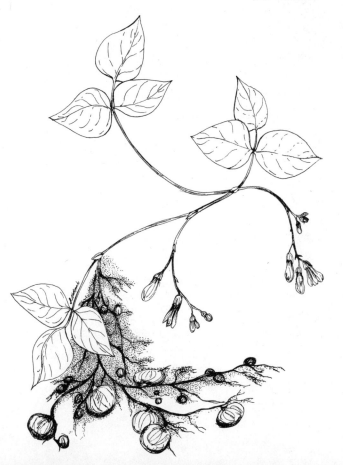

The Indians sometimes ate these beans uncooked. They removed the leathery shell by soaking the beans in warm water or in water to which hardwood ashes had been added.

The hog peanut is distributed throughout southeastern Canada to Manitoba, south to the southern United States. The underground fruits are available in late fall and early spring. These protein-rich beans are easily gathered and should be remembered, for they are an important wild-plant food.

◡§ KENTUCKY COFFEE TREE

The Pawnee and Meskwaki roasted Kentucky coffee tree seeds and ate them like nuts. Early settlers in Kentucky ground these seeds, roasted them, and used them as a coffee substitute. Although this was a fine, caffeine-free beverage, Kentucky coffee tree beans never became a popular substitute for the genuine article. Nevertheless, the large, leathery pods contain hard seeds which might be well received if they were made available by our natural-food stores.

Incidentally, the pulverized root bark used in a rectal injection was considered a sure remedy for severe cases of constipation. This effect on the bowel movement is similar to that produced in some individuals when they drink "real" coffee. Since the Kentucky coffee tree beans lack caffeine, there may be another substance that is found in both of these "coffee" plants which stimulates the bowels.

◡§ KIDNEY BEAN

The common kidney bean formed an important part of the diets of those Indian tribes of North America which cultivated at least some of their vegetable food. The bean was cultivated throughout the New World and existed in many varieties. It was known by many different Indian names, varying from one region to another.

These beans were seen in Indian corn fields by the early explorers; we learn why they were planted there from Champlain in his writings of the Indians of the Kennebec region of Maine (1605): "With this corn they put in each hill three or four Brazilian beans (*Febues du Bresil*), which are of different colors. When they grow up they interlace with the corn, which reaches to the height of from five to six feet; and they keep the ground very free from weeds."

Aside from the kidney bean, the lima bean, native to South America, was cultivated by many tribes long before the arrival of the Europeans.

The Indians ate these nutritious beans green, cooked, or dried.

WILD LICORICE

The Indians of New Mexico, Wyoming, the Northwest, and Alaska ate the sweet wild licorice roots raw or roasted them in the hot embers of a fire.

LOCUST

The gaunt locust tree, which is devoid of leaves throughout most of the year, was utilized for its seeds by the Indians. After boiling, the seeds lose their acid taste and were "much esteemed by the aborigines."

In New Mexico, the flowers of a related species of locust were eaten fresh.

The bark and roots of this common eastern tree are said to be poisonous and should be avoided, even in an emergency. The locust was widely planted as an ornamental by the early settlers and can be seen throughout the eastern states except Florida. Although the tree remains barren for many months, the foliage and flowers in their bright colors make this a highly attractive addition to the landscape.

MESQUITE (FIG. 109)

Indians of the Southwest relied heavily upon the pods of the scraggly mesquite tree. The ripe

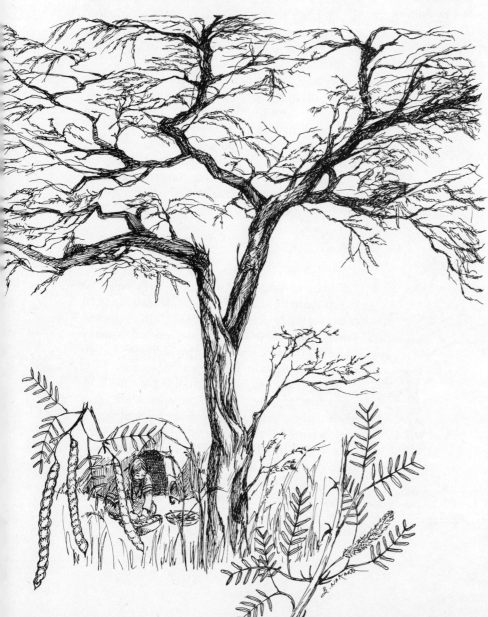

(FIG. 109) MESQUITE: *The ripe yellowish pods of this scraggly tree, which are rich in grape sugar, were eaten fresh or dried and were baked into bread by Indians of the Southwest.*

pods, which are lemon yellow, resembled string beans and still are used as food by the famished desert traveler. The pulpy, sweet substance contained in the pods is rich in grape sugar; it was eaten fresh or dried, ground, and pounded into bread and cakes which were baked in the intense desert sun.

Edward Palmer, an early anthropologist, observed this process among an unnamed tribe of the Southwest about 1870:

A female squatted herself on the ground by a wooden mortar, the lower end of which was some distance in the ground. With a long stone pestle she pounded the hard seed-pods into the meal. She then took from her head a small conical hat, and sprinkled a little water on the inside, then a little meal alternately, until the hat or bread tray was filled. After being patted on the top, it was set on the ground and exposed to the direct rays of the sun for some hours, or until it would turn out a solid cake or bread. So little water had been used to wet the meal that it seemed to me it would not stick together, but possessing a large percentage of sugar, little water was necessary. This was rather chaffy-looking bread, not unlike that made of corn meal with all the bran in it, nevertheless, it was very sweet.

The seeds too were highly valued and, like the pods, were ground into a meal and prepared as mush or porridge.

To relieve thirst and to draw some immediate sustenance from their limited environment, the desert dwellers chewed on the ripe, sweet pods in emergencies.

Although the recipe is not available, some tribes prepared *atole*, a sweet beverage, from these ground pods, or fermented the sugary pulp into beer.

The tiny, pale yellow flowers were eaten, and a delicious honey is still prepared from them. In Hawaii, up to two hundred tons of this honey were, until recently, produced and exported annually.

The inner bark contains much tannin and has been successfully utilized as a medicinal tea to arrest diarrhea. The resinous gum which appears on the bark is also rich in sugar and is edible in the raw state but is tastier when boiled into a syrup. In addition to eating it, some tribes mixed the gum with mud and applied it to their heads to rid themselves of vermin. In some cases the "mud pack" acted as a dye and temporarily colored the hair of old people "jet black."

The mesquite must not be overlooked as being an important, easily accessible survival food. When eaten raw, the sweet, lemon-tasting bean pods are highly nutritious.

The screw bean is closely related to the mesquite and utilized in the same way as an article of food. Instead of having straight or slightly curved fruits, this species has highly twisted, spiral pods which were favored by the Indians of the Colorado river region.

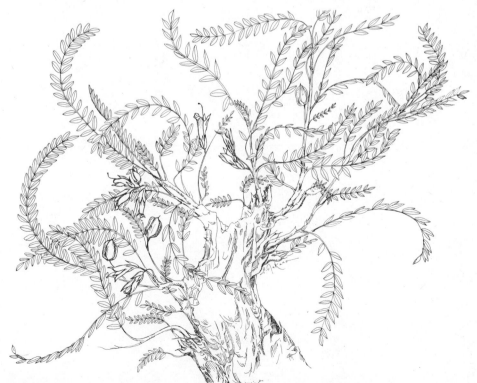

(FIG. 110) *MILK VETCH: The green fruits of this well-known plant of the prairies were eaten raw or boiled by the Indians of Montana.*

❧ MILK VETCH (GROUND PLUM)
(FIG.110)

The green, round-to-oval fruits of the well-known milk vetch of the prairies and plains were eaten raw or boiled by the Indians of Montana. Cree and Stone Indians ate the roots of a related species A. *aboriginum*; however, several species which it resembles are highly poisonous, such as the locoweed and two-grooved milk vetch.

The Zuñi collected the pods of a related milk vetch (A. *diphysus*) in the fall and ate them fresh or dried them for future use. They regarded the boiled, salted seed pods as a special treat. The Hopi also utilized the milk vetch of his environment (A. *pictus filifolius*). The roots were dug out after a rain and eaten fresh as a sweet food.

Although these plants are highly edible and readily accessible, the inexperienced plant gatherer should be careful to avoid the poisonous relatives, the locoweeds.

THE CACTI

The Indians utilized at least forty species of cacti for food or water. These desert plants were well understood, and by using special methods, the famished traveler was able to procure his essential nourishment.

Almost all cacti are edible; however, some are more nourishing or more easily approached than others. Only peyote and living rock are reportedly hallucinogenic or intoxicating. Also, one variety of the hedgehog cactus may be poisonous. The Navajos used this species as a heart stimulant, but named it *Tjeenáyookisih*, which has been translated as "plant, which if eaten makes the heart feel as if it were twisted."

In general, young cacti are tastier than older plants. The fruits, which may grow below, above, or within the cactus's flower, were the part of the plant that were most often eaten. In some cases, the pulp of the stem was pressed for its watery juice. Some tribes ate the seeds contained within the fruit of certain species, as is the case with the cottontop, the seeds of which were used by the Panamint tribe of California.

Of the three types of cacti described below, the prickly pear was the most important food-providing cactus among the Indians of the Southwest.

BARREL CACTUS (FIG.111,a)

The well-known barrel cactus is a true reservoir of water that is easily tapped. The Indians simply sliced off the top and pounded the white, pulpy interior to release the water. After withdrawing the liquid, some travelers used the hollowed plant as an oven. They simply dropped in meats and other foods, together with preheated stones, and allow them to cook.

GIANT CACTUS (SAGUARO) (FIG.111,b)

Sometimes growing to a height of forty feet, the giant cactus, or saguaro, was commonly utilized by Indians of Arizona and California. The fruits, which resemble the fig, were eaten when ripe while the rind, pulp, and seeds were sometimes dried and ground into a gruel. The Papago tribe prepared a sweet syrup by fermenting the juice from the pressed fruits. The figlike fruit is said to be "delicious, having the combined flavor of the peach, strawberry and fig."

PRICKLY PEAR (FIG.111,c)

The fleshy fruits of several of the prickly pear species, which are common to the Southwest, were important to the Indians of New Mexico, Arizona, California, and Utah. The fruits, known as *tunas*, are found beneath the flowers and are easily removed. To avoid being pricked by the large spines, the Navajo gathered the fruits with a forked branch. The Apaches used wooden tongs for the same purpose.

The skin is also studded with numerous fine downy spines which are nearly invisible to the unaided eye. To remove these, the Indians brushed the skin briskly with a bunch of grass or burned them off. Nevertheless, these barbed bristles were found in feces left by ancient Indian cultures, as examined by a contemporary anthropologist.

After gathering these fruits, the Indians sliced off the ends, sliced the fruits down one side, and dried the pulp in the sun. They were then eaten as dried fruit or preserved for use during the winter. The Pawnees cooked the dried fruit with meat or prepared a tasty applesaucelike dish with it. To make this sauce, they boiled the unripe fruit in water for ten to twelve hours and allowed it to ferment for a short while.

Some tribes prepared an emergency food from the small, fleshy leaves which grow together with the large spines. The leaves were roasted in hot ashes so that the thorns and skin could easily be removed. The "slimy, sweet, succulent substance" which remained was eaten, saving countless men from death by starvation.

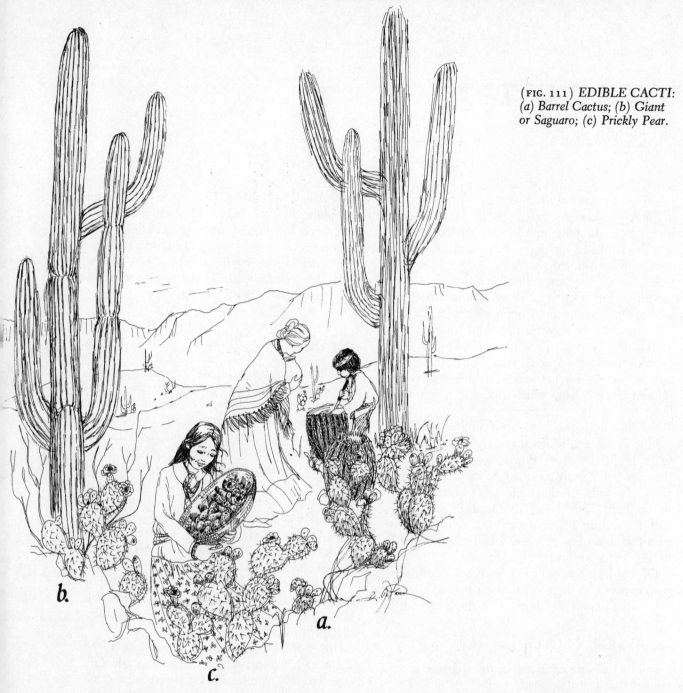

The seeds, which are easily removed from the fruit, were also utilized by the Indians. They were lightly toasted and then ground into a meal which was used to make cakes or gruel. The seeds were sometimes dried and preserved for later use.

The prickly pear has been an important plant in America since early times, and in Mexico, it is represented on the silver dollar, the state flag, and the arms of the Republic. Through Mexican folklore we learn that in 1325, the Aztecs were being pursued by a hostile people when they came upon an eagle strangling a snake atop a prickly pear. The Aztecs interpreted this as a good sign, perhaps a symbol of their eventual victory over their pursuers, and decided to settle at that site, the present location of Mexico City.

The Navajo, too, regarded these cacti in a special light. In the ceremonial sandpainting of the cactus people, four figures are drawn in the shape of these cactus plants. The laws of this tribe prohibited the use of cactus stalks for firewood. This tribe picked the fruit of the prickly pear with a caution shown no other plant. They feared that the fruit could "twist the heart;" to avoid this, they offered the plant a hair from the gatherer's head.

THE COMPOSITES
(Daisy Family)

JERUSALEM ARTICHOKE (FIG.112)

The native Jerusalem artichoke is a useful survival food because the tubers can be eaten like potatoes during the fall, winter, or spring.

The Indians ate these artichokes raw, boiled, or baked. The plant, which grew wild in the fields or along streams, was eaten as a secondary food by several tribes. Some Iroquois women became especially fond of this food and were named "artichoke eaters" by their friends.

The early settlers were quick to export this plant, and it soon became extremely popular in Europe, especially in the Mediterranean countries where the tubers were named *girasol* in Spain and *girasole* in Italy. The English evidently misinterpreted these names, changing them to

(FIG. 112) JERUSALEM ARTICHOKE: *This native plant is a useful survival food because the tubers can be eaten like potatoes during the fall, winter, or spring.*

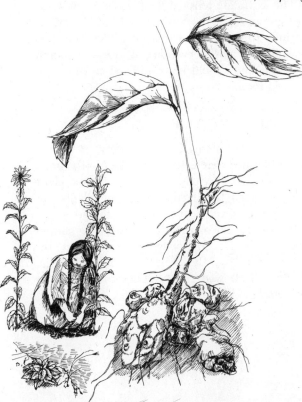

"Jerusalem." Thus the common name as it stands today.

This indigenous plant is a species of sunflower that was once extensively cultivated throughout North America. The plants have since "escaped" and are common along roadsides, in fields, or in garbage dumps. They have thick, hairy stems and grow between six and ten feet high. The bright yellow flowers bloom between July and October.

Interestingly, since these fleshy tubers reportedly lack starch, they would make a good food for people who want to avoid this carbohydrate.

LARGE-LEAVED ASTER

The young, tender leaves of the woodland large-leaved aster were eaten by the Ojibwa Indians. The Chippewas enjoyed the boiled leaves with fish.

These heart-shaped leaves are tough when mature; for this reason, only the very young plants are considered edible.

This aster blooms from July to September and has white to lavender flowerheads. It is found in dry woods in the eastern United States.

BALSAMROOT
(OREGON SUNFLOWER)

In the early spring many mountain slopes of the northwestern states and British Columbia are covered with wavy bunches of the bright yellow flowers of balsamroot. Each plant, with its thick, arrow-head-shaped leaves, may bear up to a dozen of these yellow flowers. By the time summer bears full turn, the plants have dried up and appear parched and flowerless.

The Thompson Indians of British Columbia ate the ripe seeds raw or prepared a flour from them by pounding them in a stone mortar. They sometimes boiled these rich, oily seeds with deer's fat and prepared small cakes from the mass when it had cooked.

The Indians of Puget Sound prepared a meal from the pounded seeds and baked this *mielito* into cakes.

The roots of the Oregon sunflower were cooked on hot stones by the Nez Percé Indians of Oregon and eaten with other foods. The roots have a thick crown that is edible in the uncooked state.

Easily recognized by its bright yellow flowers, this plant makes a very useful natural food.

✑ BURDOCK

The common, large-leaved, ugly-looking burdock weed is widely used as food throughout the world. Originally introduced from Europe, burdock now grows in abandoned fields and waste places throughout southern Canada and the northern states.

The Iroquois and other tribes learned from the early settlers how to prepare this weed. They dried the roots of young plants (without flowering stalks) and used them in soups. They also cooked the leaves and included them in their diet as greens.

Other portions of this backyard plant are prepared as well. In Japan, the tender young roots and leaf stalks are eaten after being boiled in two changes of water to remove the tough fibers. The young stems are also edible. They should be collected before flowering in late spring and the rind peeled before cooking. Again *two* changes of water are required.

As early as 1772, the plant was appreciated in America. Peter Kalm, the Swedish naturalist, wrote in his *Travels in North America* about a stop in Ticonderoga, New York: "and the governor told me that its tender shoots are eaten in spring as radishes, after the exterior part is taken off."

✑ SWEET COLTSFOOT

The creeping sweet coltsfoot herb, common along rivers, damp woods, and boggy meadows, provided certain tribes of northern California with a salt substitute. As Chestnut relates, this commodity was so important that it became the object of intertribal warfare:

this plant might very appropriately be called the Yuki salt plant. Hedged in from the sea by enemies, this tribe, together with the Wailakis, formerly used the ashes of various plants, but more especially of this one, for the salt which they contain, and being essentially a herbivorous people, salt was as prime a necessity for them as it is for cows and other herbivorous animals. I was told that frequent battles were fought for the possession of a certain salt supply on Stony Creek in Colusa County. To obtain the ash the stem and leaves were first rolled up into balls while still green, and after being carefully dried they were placed on top of a very small fire on a rock and burned.

✑ DANDELION

As has already been mentioned (under medicines), the roots of dandelion accounted for the saving of many lives on the island of Minorca. The leaves, best prepared by boiling in water and then chilling, are used throughout the world as greens.

Although the dandelion was introduced from Europe, many Indian tribes soon learned to enjoy eating it. The Iroquois preferred the boiled leaves with fatty meats.

Dandelion roots make an excellent coffee substitute that is free of caffeine and delicious. The roots are roasted slowly over several hours and ground when they become crisp and brown inside.

The leaves are relished by deer, while pheasants and grouse favor the seeds. In an emergency, the seedlike fruits can be eaten raw. The dandelion, available at most elevations, is rich in vitamins A and C and should be considered an important survival food.

✑ WILD LETTUCE

The leafy stems of one variety or another of wild lettuce were eaten by all the North American Indians. Since the leaves of mature plants are too tough to be enjoyed, young plants that have never flowered are preferred for greens.

In New Mexico, the Zuñis used the gum of larkspur lettuce for chewing. To obtain this "chewing gum," they cut the roots of young plants and allowed the exuding gum to dry before chewing.

☙ SAFFLOWER

The Hopi used safflower flowers to color their *piki*, or wafer bread, yellow. This "false saffron" plant was introduced to the Southwest by the Mormons, about 1870. It is cultivated in gardens which are irrigated by narrow trenches.

☙ SUNFLOWER

Wavy yellow sunflower fields hold an abundance of food that was valuable to the Indian. Long before the arrival of the European, the native American had eaten the seeds raw or roasted. The Iroquois, who probably learned of this plant from a western tribe, extracted the nutritious sunflower oil by heating the bruised, ripe seeds and then boiling the mass in water. When the oil separated from the pulp, it was allowed to cool and then skimmed off.

As a survival food, the sunflower should not be forgotten. The young flowerheads when boiled in water can be eaten like Brussels sprouts. As mentioned, the seeds can be eaten raw, and they are as much as 55 percent of readily digestible protein.

The Indians of Loretto, Canada, mixed the seeds with sagamite or corn soup, while some tribes pounded the dried kernels and used them to make cakes, bread, and soups. Some woodsmen improvise a coffeelike beverage from the roasted seeds or shells.

This plant has since been exported and has become a very important source of oil in Russia. This seems a strange fate for the state flower of Kansas.

THE FERNS

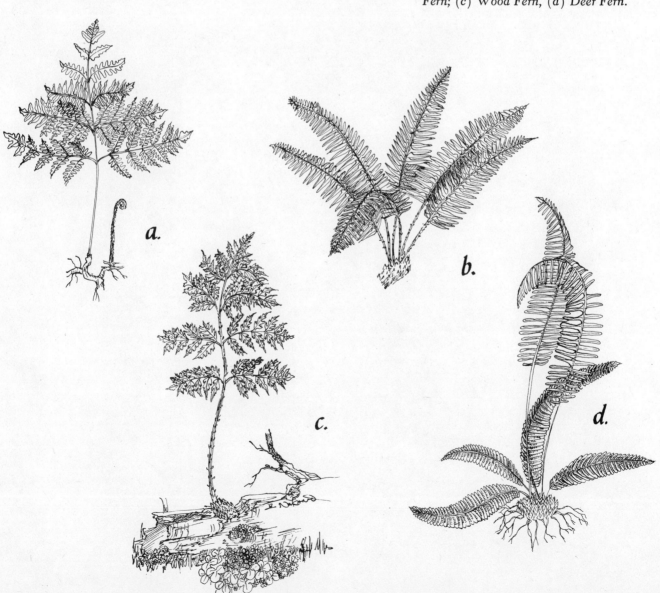

⊸§ BRACKEN (FIG.113,a)

The bracken is one of our commonest ferns; it is available as an emergency food throughout Canada and the United States. Although it is eaten on a wide scale in New Zealand and Japan, the bracken has not yet been popularly accepted in America. Nevertheless, several Indian tribes utilized this fern as a green vegetable and in making bread.

Only the young plants, less than eight inches tall, were eaten because the older, dry brackens are terrible to taste. This is fortunate because the full-grown fronds are slightly toxic and have been responsible for poisoning grazing stock.

The Indians sometimes ate the young, uncoiled sprouts raw, as during a hunt as reported by H. H. Smith:

Hunters are very careful to live wholly upon this when stalking does in the spring. The doe feeds

(FIG. 113) *COMMON EDIBLE FERNS: (a) Bracken; (b) Sword Fern; (c) Wood Fern, (d) Deer Fern.*

a.

b.

c.

d.

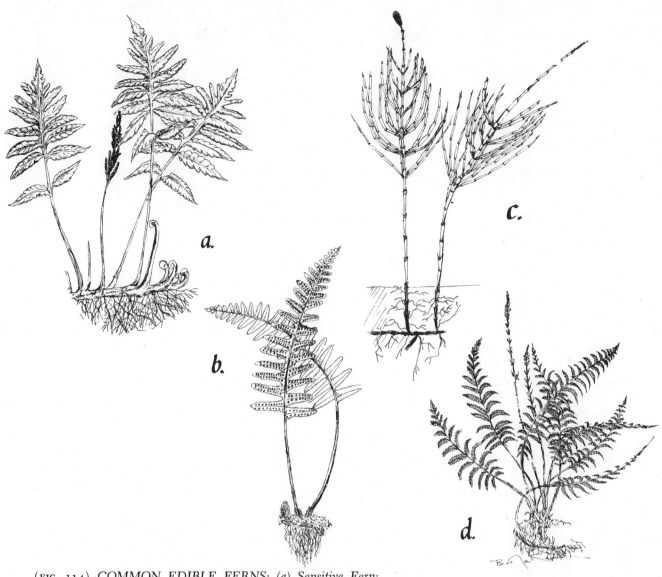

(FIG. 114) COMMON EDIBLE FERNS: (a) Sensitive Fern;
(b) California Polypody; (c) Horsetail; (d) Cinnamon Fern.

upon the fronds and the hunter does also, so that his breath does not betray his presence. He claims to be able to approach within 20 feet without disturbing the deer, from which distance he can easily make a fatal shot with his bow and arrow.

Some tribes boiled the young sprouts in water to obtain an oil and starch.

Some outdoors cookbooks call for a similar preparation, and recommend that the young, thicker stalks be selected, the curled tops and bases removed, and the stalks then boiled in salted water for thirty to sixty minutes or until tender. They are described as a delicious asparaguslike vegetable that is especially tasty with added salt, pepper, and melted butter.

Many tribes also used the rhizomes as an im-portant food. The white center was baked in hot embers until it became soft and doughy. This pulp was then eaten or stored for future use. Bread was also made from the dried, pulverized rhizomes.

Bracken, which has been eaten in many countries in times of scarcity, should be considered a useful survival food. The uncurled fronds are used in soups while the ground roots have often provided bread for the starving.

Bracken was by far the most valuable of the edible ferns so far as Indian use is concerned. In some cases it was a major constituent of a tribe's sustenance. Other ferns which were used as food include the cinnamon fern. The Menominees boiled the fronds of these young plants and used them to thicken soups.

CALIFORNIA POLYPODY (FIG.114,b)

An early writer reported that the California polypody rhizome was eaten as a food staple by the "Sierra Indians."

DEER FERN (FIG.113,d)

In California, deer fern fronds were eaten as food in emergencies or to alleviate thirst on long journeys.

HORSETAIL FERN (FIG.114,c)

In New Mexico, the Hopi Indians mixed the dried, ground stems of *E. laevigatum* the horsetail fern with corn meal and ate it as a mush or baked it as bread. The Lower Chinook Indians of Washington ate the peeled, raw stems of young shoots of the field horsetail, while the Cowlitz tribe, of the same region, cooked portions of the root stalk of the giant horsetail as food.

In emergencies the horsetails might be considered as survival foods; however, some authors consider certain varieties poisonous to livestock. For this reason most wilderness recipes suggest that the young reproductive shoots be boiled for about twenty minutes in each of three or four waters.

SENSITIVE FERN (FIG.114,a)

The Iroquois Indians utilized the rhizomes of the sensitive fern in times of scarcity. Also known as fiddleheads, these ferns have been sold in vegetable markets in the East as delicacies. One commercial recipe calls for removing the brown scales and then steaming them in very little water. In an emergency, practically any succulent, young unopened frond, or fiddlehead, could be eaten.

SWORD FERN (FIG.113,b)

In Washington, the Indians peeled the fleshy rhizomes of sword fern and baked them like potatoes with salmon eggs in pit ovens. Berries were sometimes placed on the fronds to dry.

WOOD FERN (FIG.113,c)

Alaskan and Californian natives dug wood fern rhizomes in spring and baked them in stone earth ovens.

THE GOOSEFOOT FAMILY

The goosefoot family, which includes spinach and beets, does not contain any native food plants which were of major importance to the Indians. Nevertheless, the following species provided flavoring, greens, and a seed flour.

GLASSWORT (FIG.115,a)

The Indians of Utah and Nevada gathered the seeds of the fleshy herb glasswort and ground them to flour, which was used in various ways.

These plants are common in salt marshes, and a related European variety has long been used as a pickle plant or as a salad. To make these pickles, the stems and branches were first boiled in salt water and then soaked in vinegar.

The plants received their common name by virtue of the high soda content of several species which made them valuable in the manufacture of glass and soap. Glasswort ashes are known as *barilla* in these industries.

LAMB'S-QUARTERS (PIGWEED) (FIG.115,b)

The young leaves of the common weed lamb's-quarters were eaten as greens or boiled with fat by many tribes. It is found in nearly all gardens and makes an excellent wild spinach which is sweeter to the taste than market spinach.

The tiny, hard seeds were also utilized as a wild food. They are generally ground into meal and baked as bread or added to corn meal for similar baked goods.

These common plants are readily available and should not be overlooked for their tender, tasty stems and leaves. It is reported that during times of scarcity, Napoleon lived on the black bread made from seeds of pigweed.

SALTBUSH (FIG.115,c)

Like the pigweed, the annual saltbush herb is very common along the seashores of both

(FIG. 115) (a) GLASS-WORT: *The seeds of this common dweller of salt marshes were ground into flour by Indians of Utah and Nevada; (b) PIGWEED: The young leaves of this common weed were eaten as greens or boiled with fat by many tribes; (c) SALT-BUSH: The saltbushes occur in the vicinity of dry lakes or in salt marshes. The stems and leaves were boiled with other foods while the seeds were ground into flour; (d) SEA BLITE: Indians of the Southeast and West boiled the leaves and ate them as greens or ground the seeds into flour.*

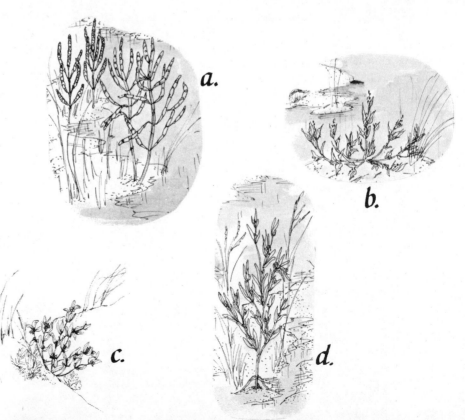

a.

b.

c.

d.

coasts of America; it makes excellent greens or "spinach." The Indians availed themselves of the stems and leaves by boiling them with other foods, while some tribes used the water in which they were boiled on corn pudding. The seeds, very naturally, were ground into flour that was used for thin porridge or bread.

The saltbushes typically occur in salt marshes or in the vicinity of dry lakes; however, several inland varieties appear in the rich soil of waste places throughout the continent. These plants are not extremely interesting to look at, but like the other members of the goosefoot family, they should be learned for the excellent foods they provide.

SEA BLITE (FIG.115,d)

Indians of the Southeast and West boiled the leaves of the sea blites and ate them as greens or ground the seeds into flour.

They inhabit the same alkaline environments as the other plants listed under this family and would make a useful survival food. Several wilderness writers recommend that the leaves, when cooked, be boiled in two or three changes of water to eliminate their excessive salt content.

THE GRASSES

✑ BARLEY

The seeds of several species of barley were used by Indians in Utah, Nevada, Oregon, and California. Aside from making the common parched seed flour, some tribes made a coffee substitute from the singed seed coats.

✑ CALIFORNIA BROME

The rough, hairy California brome grass, known as poverty grass by the early settlers, was used for its heavy seeds by the Indians. These seeds were parched and then ground into meal that is commonly known as *piñole*, a Spanish word that is universally applied to *any* meal derived from parched seeds.

✑ SOUTHERN CANE

Southern cane is common to the region south of Virginia and Kentucky. As E. L. Sturtevant points out, "It produces an abundant crop of seed with heads very like those of broom corn.

The seeds are . . . said to be not much inferior to wheat, for which the Indians and occasionally the first settlers substituted it."

✑ MAIZE (INDIAN CORN) (FIG.116)

Cultivated maize is the Indian's greatest contributor to the world's food resources. Maize was eaten throughout much of North America and is thought to have originated in Mexico, from wild corn.

In ancient times the Indian expended most of his energy hunting and seeking wild plant foods. It was only with the coming of agriculture, when corn fields and vegetable gardens began to provide sufficient food, that small bands of Indians grew into communities. Once nomadic, they slowly came to enjoy a leisure time. As the early, small varieties of corn increased in size, the importance of this food crop also grew until it became the center of the art and religious life of many tribes. Countless ceremonies were performed for this food, so that by the time the

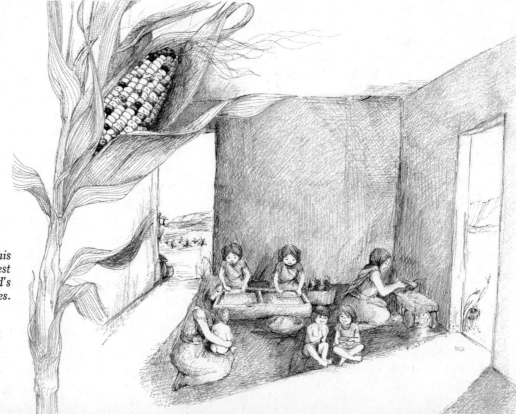

(FIG. 116) MAIZE: *This plant is the Indian's greatest contribution to the world's food resources.*

Europeans arrived, some tribes referred to maize by words which mean "our life" or "it sustains us" or "giver of life." New cultures originated with the introduction of this crop.

Corn is a highly nutritious food, some varieties being more than 12 percent protein. Every tribe that cultivated maize developed their own recipes and rituals for preparing it. No doubt, some interchange between tribes, and between the Indians and whites, accounts for the universal recipes, such as hominy or leaf cakes from green corn.

The corn preparations described below are only a few of many which are available in numerous reference works, especially in the *Iroquois Use of Maize and Other Food Plants* by Arthur C. Parker.

1. Leaf cakes: This recipe was important among the Iroquois and the Navajo, while among the Zuñi it was considered "makeshift." The general procedure follows: Kernels of green corn were removed from the cob and beaten to a paste between stones. This mass was then divided into small cakes, each of them wrapped tightly with green corn leaves. The secured masses were then boiled in water for forty-five minutes, or covered with moist earth and then baked in hot coals for one hour. The charred leaf jackets were removed and the cakes eaten with bear fat or sunflower oil or dried in the sun and stored for winter use when it was boiled with meat or steamed and eaten with salt.

2. Hominy: This was a food staple of the Zuñi Indians. Kernels of corn were boiled in a mixture of water and wood ashes and then stirred. This mixture was boiled for three hours, being stirred throughout, after which time the corn was removed to a basket and rinsed in a flowing stream. The pulpy corn meal was then boiled in water with meat and beans which were added for flavor.

3. Popped corn: The ripe kernels were simply toasted in pottery on the hot stones of a fire and stirred until they popped. They were eaten while hot, with salt.

4. Paper bread: Corn was crushed between stones, toasted as in popped corn and stirred constantly to prevent burning, and ground twice again. This meal was then mixed with cold water and then boiled. When cool, the batter was cooked on a hot stone slab which had been oiled with pulverized watermelon or squash seeds. By the time the thin batter had been spread across the hot slab, it was already cooked. This wafer bread was sometimes colored with various natural dyes. Since it was very light, the Indians often carried it as a food staple during long expeditions.

5. Batter husks: The Zuñi had a novel recipe which called for the labor of several young girls to chew corn meal for the purpose of converting the starch to sugar, thereby sweetening the end product. "As each girl finds it necessary she ejects the meal into a small bowl. . . . Dried corn husks are dampened. . . . and the batter is spread over them." The husks were then cooked overnight and eaten the following morning.

6. Corn beverages: The Zuñi prepared "bead water" by grinding popped corn into a fine powder and then adding it to cold water. After straining, the mixture was drunk, especially by the priests during ceremonies.

The same tribe made a fermented beverage by exposing dampened kernels to the sun until they sprouted. These sprouts were then left to stand in water for a few days and then drunk.

The Iroquois prepared a "corn coffee" by parching dried ears of corn on hot embers and then scraping the kernels into a container. Boiling water was added and the mixture again boiled for about five minutes, when the "coffee" was ready for drinking with maple sugar added as a sweetener.

✑ DARNEL

There is much controversy as to whether the darnel grass is poisonous. By V. K. Chestnut's account, it appears as if the parable "what you don't know won't hurt you" is true. Both the Little Lake and Yuki Indians ate the seeds for pinole without ill effects. Those who hold that Darnel is dangerous state that its poisonous qualities are due to the presence of a fungus on the grain. Chestnut offers one explanation for the California tribes' apparent immunity to this poison fungus: "It seems probable that the grain is not poisonous in this locality, but it is possible that the poison is destroyed in the process of parching."

BARNYARD GRASS (FIG.117)

The coarse, broad-leaved barnyard grass has good-sized seeds which were eaten by many tribes. The seeds are available from early July to September, but must be gathered before they become too ripe. They are simply prepared, Indian style, by parching and grinding between stones. This flour was mixed with milk or water and baked into the usual products.

All grasses produce edible seeds that could be parched and eaten in emergencies. Care should be taken to avoid gathering the poisonous fungus, ergot, which may appear as a small, dark body in place of the grass seed.

(FIG. 117) BARNYARD GRASS: *The seeds of this coarse grass were eaten by many tribes. They were simply parched, ground between stones, and baked.*

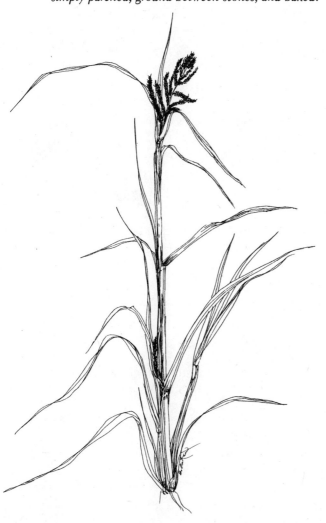

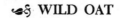 ### WILD OAT

Wild oat, which resembles the cultivated variety, was commonly used by the Indians of California. The tough, sharply pointed seeds were thrown together with hot coals and shaken in a basket that was specially made to withstand the heat. The parched seed was then ground in a stone mortar until the desired flour was formed. The Pomos of northern California ate this flour in the raw, uncooked state, with a little salt added for flavor.

INDIAN MOUNTAIN-RICE (FIG.118)

The tufted grass Indian mountain-rice contains rather large seeds which were used as food staples by at least one tribe of the Southwest

(FIG. 118) INDIAN MOUNTAIN-RICE: *The Zuñi Indians sought the large seeds of this tufted grass when their farm crops failed.*

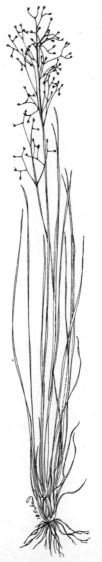

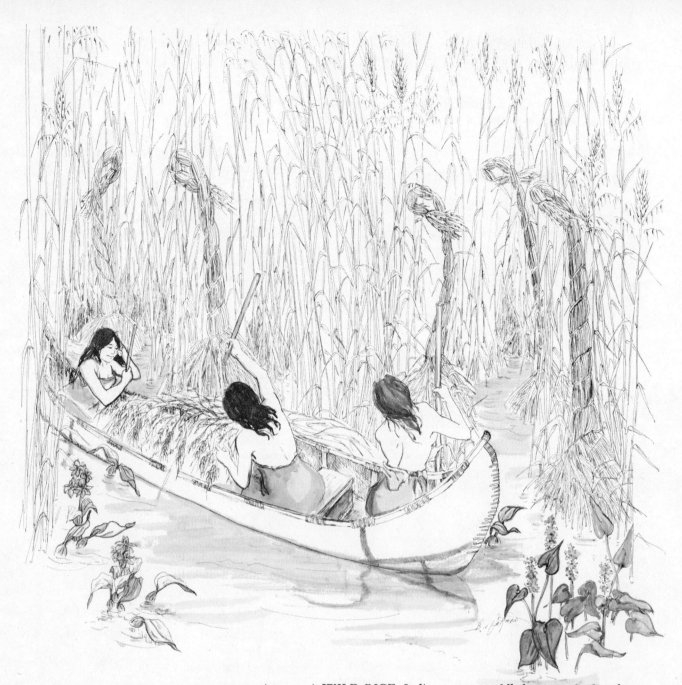

(FIG. 119) WILD RICE: *Indian women paddled among the bunches of bound rice plants beating the ripened seeds into their canoes.*

before corn was introduced from Mexico. An early anthropologist, Palmer, reported that the Zuñi Indians "when their farm crops fail, become wandering hunters after the seeds of this grass. . . . Parties are sometimes seen ten miles from their villages, on foot, carrying enormous loads for winter provision."

The Indians parched the seeds over a fire to remove the fine hairs. They are easily ground into flour and can be cooked into cakes or added to soups. Mountain-rice seeds are about 6 percent sugars and 20 percent starch.

An eastern variety, *O. asperifolia*, is found in dry woods from Newfoundland to New York. It contains even larger seeds which are said to make an excellent flour.

WILD RICE (FIG.119)

The large, plume-topped grass wild rice is found growing in ponds and swamps and along the marshy borders of streams throughout the central and eastern states. The seeds were a very important cereal food among the Ojibwa and Chippewa Indians. The Menominee tribe was even named for their dependence upon this wild food. They called themselves *Menomin*, or "Wild Rice Men," because they lived mainly on the wild rice of the lakes of their region.

Indian women did the rice gathering. Before the rice was ripe, they paddled among the bunches, binding several tall rice plants together every few feet. The women returned to the rice on the day of ripening and collected the ripened grain by bending the bound shocks over their canoes and beating them with a stick. Whatever few grains fell outside of their canoes became the next generation of rice and was gathered during the next season of collection.

The Indians prepared wild rice by parching the seeds in a receptacle for a short while over hot coals. The rice was stirred constantly to keep from burning. When cool, the husks were beaten off and the seeds winnowed. The parched seeds were then boiled in water and eaten with blueberries or maple syrup or used for thickening soups. Like the commercial variety, wild rice swells with boiling, sometimes increasing in size from three to four times during cooking.

The Indians recognized the high food value of this species and many ceremonies were devoted to the cult of the wild rice plant. The Menominees held a yearly thanksgiving festival when the Great Manitou was thanked for providing this food for his people. This ceremony is held just after the rice has been gathered and before the fall hunts begin.

BEARDLESS WILD RYE

Beardless wild rye, a tall, grayish green grass which is very common to the meadows and hills of Round Valley in Mendocino County, was one of the primary sources of seed used for piñole. Also known as wild wheat, it "makes an excellent fodder after most other grasses have been dried up in late summer."

WHEAT (FIG.120)

Wheat was introduced to the Indians of the Southwest by the Spaniards. To the island of St. Croix, Maine, the French introduced wheat in 1604. The Western Company introduced wheat into the Mississippi Valley in 1718.

The Zuñis made turnovers of wheat and added sour dough to raise the mixture. An early eth-

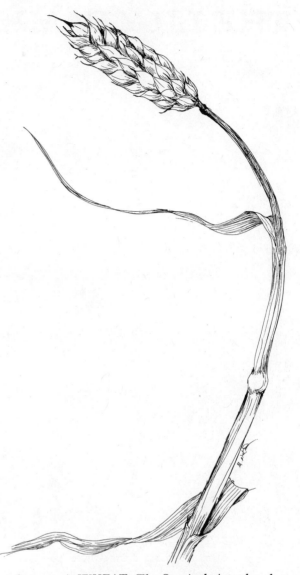

(FIG. 120) WHEAT: *The Spaniards introduced wheat to the Indians of the Southwest.*

nologist describes how old Zuñi women took great joy in shaping wheat batter into "obscene figures" prior to baking them.

M. C. Stevenson, the ethnologist, describes the Zuñi methods for making doughnuts, as adopted from the Mexicans:

A soft dough is made of flour and cold water, and salt is added. A bit of the dough broken from the mass is shaped into a cake about 4 by 4 inches. The cakes are cooked in boiling beef fat or mutton grease, or in lard. . . . Each doughnut is punched with a slender stick which is employed to turn it over in the grease and to remove it from the pot.

THE LILY FAMILY

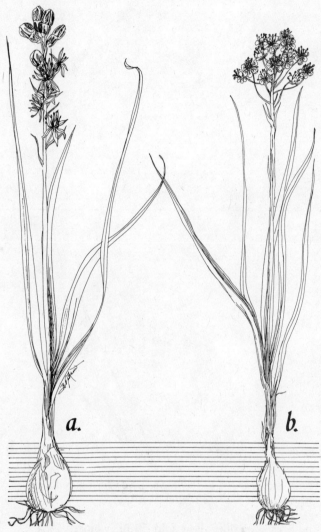

(FIG. 121) (a) COMMON CAMASS: Many intertribal wars were fought by Indians of the Northwest over the rights to collect these bulbs. Camass bulbs were eaten fresh or were baked in pits beneath several layers of pine needles; (b) DEATH CAMASS: This plant was often mistaken for the edible camass and has caused severe poisoning and even death. The edible camass has blue flowers whereas the dangerous camass has white- to cream-colored flowers.

ASPARAGUS

The well-known asparagus is listed here to exemplify that most members of this family are not lilies at all. This large group is made up of over three thousand species, many of which are garden or house plants or eaten as food.

Introduced from Europe, it was soon adopted by the Iroquois who boiled the stalks and ate them as greens.

Wild asparagus is occasionally found throughout the United States, and its seeds are sometimes roasted and ground, and then used as a substitute for coffee. We are warned by one author that they may be poisonous.

COMMON CAMASS (FIG.121,a)

The bulbs of the common camass formed such an important part of the food of the Indians of the Northwest that many intertribal wars were fought over the rights to collect them. One writer considers this plant the source of the "most widely used food roots of the Indians."

The most general method of cooking these bulbs was by baking them in pits, as described by V. K. Chestnut:

Several families get together in the evening with their supply of the bulbs. A hole of appropriate size is dug in the ground and lined with stones. A fire is then built in the hole and after it has died down the ashes are thickly covered with pine needles. The bulbs are spread upon this, another thick layer of pine needles is added, and the hole is well covered with dirt. A small fire is kept burning over the hole for the remainder of the night and all next day, when the bulbs are removed and divided among the owners.

The bulbs were then eaten or dried for storage. In British Columbia they were sometimes mixed with *Alectoria jubata*, "a dark thread-like lichen." The bulbs are low in starch content but contain a great deal of sugar and taste sweet after cooking.

Camass bulbs eaten in the fresh, uncooked state are said to be almost tasteless but crisp and mucilagenous. These bulbs were generally gathered during the flowering period of the plant, between June and July, because the deadly death camass (FIG.121,b) looks especially similar during the seasons when they both lack flowers. The common camass, which is edible as described, has *blue* flowers, while the death camass has *white* to *cream*-colored ones. The dangerous species was often mistakenly gathered along with wild onions and has caused severe poisoning and even death. The novice plant collector should be very careful with these plants.

◄§ DOGTOOTH VIOLET

Dogtooth violets are beautiful plants that are easily recognized by the two or three oblong leaves surrounding a single flower stalk which bears from one to several flowers. In the East, the yellow adder's tongue bears a single yellow, bell-shaped lily. The bulbs of both species are edible; however, the plants are too beautiful and too scarce to be gathered indiscriminately. They should be eaten only in emergencies.

◄§ LILIES

All of our native species of lilies are edible and were eaten raw or cooked in soups. The four most commonly eaten lilies are the Columbia lily and the panther lily, both native to the Northwest, the orangecup lily of the northcentral states, and the Turk's-cap lily, which was described by Thoreau as being cooked in soups by the Indians of Maine.

◄§ MARIPOSA AND SEGO LILIES
(FIG.122)

The small bulbs of the mariposa and sego lilies were important to the Indians, who ate them raw or roasted them in the embers of a fire. The sweet bulbs of these lilies saved the lives of early Mormons whose crops were devastated by locusts in 1848.

Some tribes pounded the dried bulbs into a

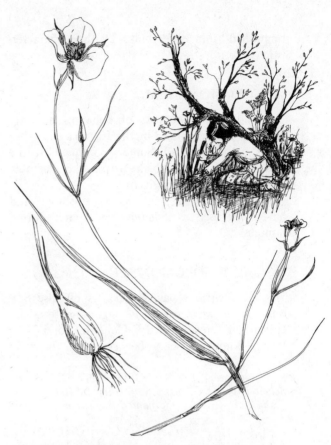

(FIG. 122) MARIPOSA LILY: *These sweet bulbs saved the lives of early Mormon settlers whose crops had been devastated by locusts in 1848.*

flour and used it for porridge or mush. The bulbs can be stored for long periods of time.

◄§ WILD ONIONS, GARLICS, AND LEEKS

The Menominee tribe named a region that was rich in the strong-smelling wild leeks *shika'ko* or skunk place. This has become *Chicago* in English. The original location of the strong-smelling bulbs has been buried beneath stockyards, highways, and apartment houses.

Wild onions, garlics, and leeks have been used for their edible bulbs since ancient times, both in the Old World and in America.

The Indians simply ate the bulbs raw or cooked them with other foods for flavor, just as we use them today. The Iroquois boiled meadow garlics, seasoned them with oil, and ate them along with other foods.

These vegetables are readily available in the wild state across North America and may be distinguished from other bulbs by their characteristic odor.

SOLOMON'S-SEAL

The thick rootstocks of Solomon's-seal are edible and were utilized by the Iroquois and other tribes to make bread. Some woodsmen eat the tender new shoots—which are said to resemble asparagus in taste—as greens.

Varieties of this plant occur in Europe and have been used as a major food source during famines.

FALSE SOLOMON'S-SEAL (FIG.123)

The delicious pale red berries of false Solomon's-seal were eaten in large quantities by Indians of Oregon, British Columbia, and Wisconsin. Known as scurvy-berries among the early

(FIG. 123) *FALSE SOLOMON'S-SEAL: The delicious pale red berries were eaten by Indians and the early settlers, who named them scurvy berries.*

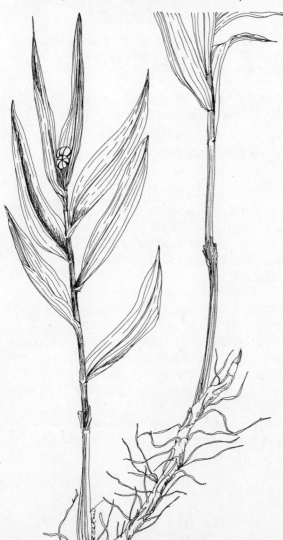

settlers, these juicy fruits were probably eaten for their vitamin C.

The Ojibwa tribe prepared the rootstocks in the same way as potatoes. To rid them of their bitter taste they were first soaked in ashes which had been mixed in water and then boiled for a short while to eliminate the "lye."

The young shoots are sometimes used as a substitute for asparagus.

This large member of the lily family bears alternate oval leaves and sometimes grows to a height of three feet. From May to July it blooms a large terminal cluster of greenish white flowers. These are followed by berries which stand out in autumn when other plants are losing their foliage. False Solomon's-seal prefers shaded woods and streamsides and is found throughout southern Canada and North America south to Georgia, Arizona, and Missouri.

YUCCA (FIG.124)

Yucca plants were extremely useful to Indians of the Southwest. The fruits of the datil

(FIG. 124) *YUCCA: The dried fruit of this plant, grass seeds, and venison were the chief foods of the early Navajo warriors when they journeyed over great distances.*

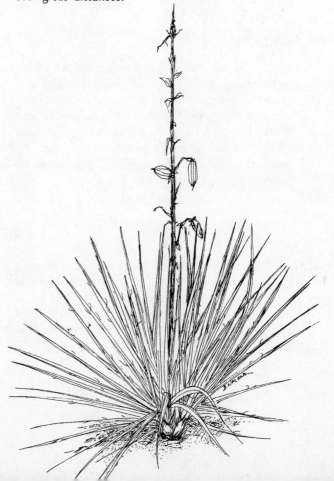

yucca, or spanish bayonet, were split open, the seeds removed, and dried in the sun. This dried fruit, along with grass seeds and venison, was the chief food of the early Navajo warriors when they journeyed over great distances. The fruits were sometimes baked on hot coals or stones and then ground and made into cakes which were used in gruel, bread, soups, etc.

The Apaches and other tribes boiled the older flowers or ate them raw.

In addition to their use as food, some of the yuccas were used for their leaf fibers. The leaves were soaked in water until soft and then pounded until the tough fibers loosened. They were then twined into cordage about the sharp center rib of the leaf. This was used for mats, cords, baskets, etc. The roots were sometimes crushed and used for soap. This natural cleanser was highly prized by the Indians, especially the Hopi who, as A. F. Whiting has reported, also used it as a hair restorer. As one of his informants related: "To cure baldness, which is very rare, wash the hair with yucca root and rub with duck grease, because ducks have such heavy feathers."

Yucca was used on the treeless plains to make fire drills. The Teton Dakota tied the hard, pointed leaf tips together as the drill and used the dried, peeled stem as the base of the fire drill.

THE MAPLES

The Maples (FIG.125) were venerated by the Iroquois and other tribes of the northern United States and southern Canada. Maple sap was drunk fresh from the tree or fermented into an intoxicating beverage. To produce a vinegar which was later sweetened with maple sugar and poured over broiled venison, the Potawatomi Indian simply allowed the fermenting process to continue for a long time.

To withdraw the sap from the tree, the Indian made a vertical slash about two inches deep and one foot long, starting about four feet from the ground. He then drove a flat stick into the lower end of the cut, and as the sap was driven up the tree by pressure, it ran over the stick into a bark trough.

Sugar was prepared from maple sap by adding heated stones to the liquid until it boiled. The resulting syrup was then strained. Another method was simpler: The sap was allowed to freeze overnight; the next day the ice was chipped off, leaving the syrup in the trough.

Maple sugar, or syrup, was mixed with pulverized corn and taken as a highly nutritious food on long journeys. It was sometimes used as a sauce which was cooked into roasting meats. The Iroquois carried maple syrup on journeys in empty quail and duck eggs. These eggs were probably the first "no-deposit–no-return" containers, but they were biodegradable and not a source of permanent litter.

Several tribes used the dried inner bark of the maples for making bread. The bark was pounded between stones, sifted to remove slivers of wood or other rough fibers, and baked in stone ovens.

Other parts of these great trees are also edible. The large seeds are boiled, with the wings removed, and eaten hot, while maple seedlings gathered in early spring are eaten fresh or dried for future use.

Several varieties of maple were used by the Indians for food. The Crow Indians made sugar from the sap of the box elder or ash-leaved maple. In central Canada this tree was widely used for its sap and early experiments indicated that the box elder produced more sap than any other maple. As with all sap-producing trees, a sunny day which followed a freezing night is best for collecting sap—the alternate cold and heat contracting and then expanding the wood drives the sap through the drainage holes. Box elder is common in the Middle West and is readily found in Chicago, Denver, and Dallas. It is the only maple with leaves composed of three leaflets, but it bears typical maple seeds with wings.

Although the sugar derived from the red maple is considered inferior to that of the sugar maple, this tree was also used for its sap by certain Indian groups. The red maple is one of our most beautiful native trees, showing red somewhere on its boughs throughout the year.

Silver maple yields a sugar of good quality, but the yield is usually 50 percent less than that of the sugar maple. Indians of the northern states used the sap for sugar and for flavoring foods, and some writers considered it to be the sweetest of all maples.

The sugar maple is considered by some to be the most beautiful tree in the world. The Iroquois would probably agree, for this species provided them with sustenance; they considered it a "special gift of the Creator." Although this tribe valued all forest trees, the sugar maple was worshipped each spring at the Maple Thanksgiving ceremony as the sign of a new year. "Its returning and rising sap . . . was the sign of the Creator's renewed covenant."

The sugar maple is the most prolific producer of all, some orchards having trees which averaged four gallons of sap with "yields as high as thirty-three pounds from a single tree." Sturtevant continues, as he relates the importance of this tree to tribes of the Midwest:

In 1870, the Winnebagoes and Chippewas are said often to sell to the Northwest Fur Company fifteen thousand pounds of sugar a year. The sugar season among the Indians is a sort of carnival, and boiling candy and pouring it out on the snow to cool is the pastime of the children.

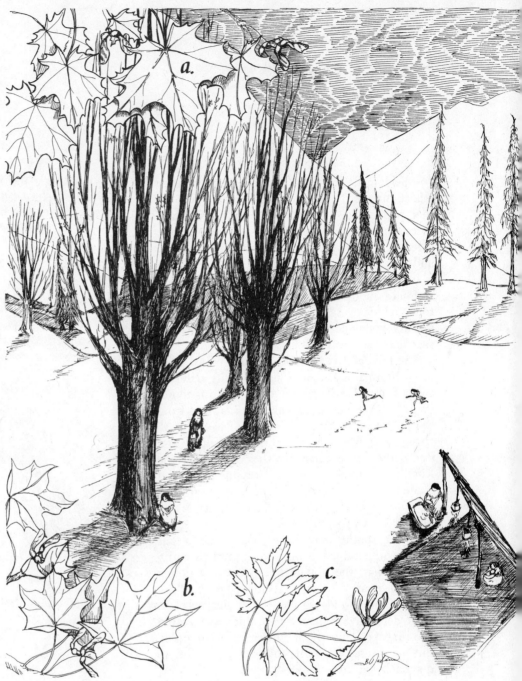

Maple sugar, incidentally, could provide a sweetener for the natural food purists who avoid either white "refined" sugar or "brown" sugar, which is simply white sugar with molasses added for coloring. When maple sap is heated for a few hours at a low temperature to avoid scorching, the original volume is greatly reduced and the dark, granular mass that remains makes a fine natural sweetener.

Although maple beer was not an Indian recipe it is included here, as described by M. L. Fernald and A. C. Kinsey (from Michaux) for those innovative spirits who are not purists: "Upon 4 gallons of boiling water, pour 1 quart of Maple molasses [syrup]; add a little yeast or leaven to excite the fermentation, and a spoonful of the essence of spruce: a very pleasant and salutary drink is thus obtained."

THE PALMS

Seldom do we think of the palms when we reflect on the North American Indian and his food plants. Nevertheless, the delicious fruits and cores of leaves and stems of several palms were eaten in season by tribes of the southern Atlantic and lower Pacific coasts.

In southern California, the blue palm, which is found in desert canyons, was sought for its round, brown, sweet fruits. In times of food scarcity young leaves were torn open and their succulent bases eaten.

The fan palm (FIG. 126), the only native palm of California, was also sought for its datelike, sweet fruits. This large interesting palm is found in groves around springs and moist areas from southern California to Arizona and Mexico. Although the black or brown fruits are hard and small, they were eaten for their sweetness; the leaf buds and seeds were ground into meal and made into bread, gruel, etc. The leaves were used to some extent for roofs and baskets while the fiber was used for making cord.

In the southeastern states, the palmetto was of such importance to the Indians and the early settlers that the founders of South Carolina adopted it as their state symbol. These palms, native from Florida to North Carolina, were in great demand for their cores, which were eaten like cabbage. An early chronicler (1613) recorded the many uses to which this palm was put, as quoted by Sturtevant:

> There is a tree called a Palmito tree, which hath a very sweet berry, upon which the hogs doe most feede; but our men, finding the sweetnesse of them, did willingly share with the hogs for them, they being very pleasant and wholesome, which made them carelesse almost of any bread with their meate . . . take a hatchet and cut him [the tree], or an augur and bore him, and it yields a very pleasant liquor, much like unto your sweete wines.

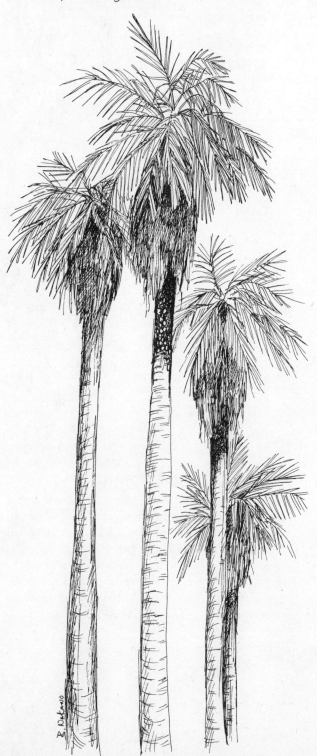

(FIG. 126) FAN PALM: *This native of California was sought for its datelike, sweet fruits. The leaves were used for roofs and baskets, while the fiber was used for making cord.*

THE PARSLEY FAMILY

The parsley family contains many vegetables that are well known to us and that were eaten by the native American. These include angelica, the fresh, new sprouts of which were eaten raw and the roots of which were boiled; anise, which was used as a spice on pinole; carrots; celery; coriander, the leaves of which were eaten fresh and the roots of which were pulverized and used as a flavoring with meat; parsley; and the parsnip.

The highly poisonous water hemlock belongs to this family and resembles several of the edible plants listed above. Each season many cows and sheep die as a result of eating this species; the inexperienced food gatherer should learn its characteristics. In Oregon, the Klamath Indians prepared poison-tipped arrows from a mixture of rotted deer's liver, the venom of a rattlesnake, and the juice of this plant.

Only a few members of the parsley family were of great food value to the Indians; these will be discussed below.

✍ BISCUIT ROOT

Biscuit root was another of the Indians' favorite root foods. The writings of nearly all the early explorers refer to this plant by the antiquated popular names, couse, or kouse. These closely related species grow abundantly west of the Rocky Mountains and were gathered mainly for their roots, although some tribes made a beverage by boiling the flowers, stems, and leaves.

The small roots were eaten raw or pounded into large cakes which were dried in the sun prior to cooking. They were sometimes stored for use during winter and obviously kept very well.

The young sprouts and leaves make excellent greens and were used for this purpose by the Indians of California and British Columbia. This plant generally inhabits dry prairies and hillsides and is an excellent emergency food.

✍ COW PARSNIP

The young, tender leaf and flower stalks of the cow parsnip were commonly eaten raw by tribes across North America, north to Alaska. The roots were also eaten, after boiling.

To render the stems palatable they are peeled and boiled in two waters. They taste like cooked celery and are highly nutritious, containing about 18 percent protein. Of course, the stems are edible raw—Indian style—and may be thinly sliced and

(FIG. 127) YAMPA: *The Indians of Colorado considered this the best of all root foods. This plant was of such importance that in northwestern Colorado a valley, river, and town are named for it.*

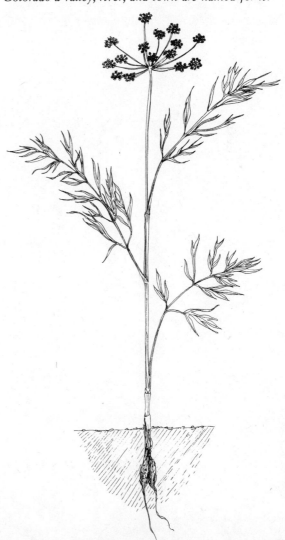

eaten in salads. Some people even eat the leaves, fresh or cooked.

This easily recognized plant is found in moist soil, almost with the distribution of a weed, across southern Canada and all of the United States. It is readily gathered and an excellent survival food.

✑§ YAMPA (FIG.127)

Yampa was considered the best of all root foods among the Indians of Colorado. The plant grows in abundance in the region of the Yampa River in northwestern Colorado, and as Harrington points out, it was of such importance in that location that a valley, river, and town were named for it.

These small roots are very tasty and were either eaten raw, boiled, roasted, or dried. They are found throughout the Rocky Mountain States, north to Canada, and would be good to learn as a food item.

Very often wars have originated over competition for food supplies. The Shoshoni were forced to attack stage coaches and the pony express when their grass and root foods were ravaged by the cattle and sheep which had been brought in by prospectors after the discovery of the Comstock Lode. No doubt yampa was one of these ravaged wild plants.

THE PINE FAMILY

The pines were one of the most frequently used families of edible plants. Although nearly all pine seeds are edible, the pines of the West contain much larger and more delicious seeds than any of the eastern varieties. The inner bark of all species is edible and has saved many souls from starvation. This sap-filled inner layer was so frequently employed as an emergency food and for a "flour" that great stands of these trees were found stripped of their bark by early explorers in North America.

The Mohawk name *Adirhōn'dak* describes a group of Indians who were "tree eaters." They ate quantities of the inner bark of the tops of pines, "especially in the spring when it was full of sweet sap."

Although each type of edible pine will be treated below, the Zuñi method of preparing bread from the inner bark is worth describing for it is a general method which can be applied to any of these species.

Zuñi women first removed the rough outer bark and gathered the young inner layer by scraping with a sharpened stone or animal horn. Next, the inner bark was boiled and pounded into a mash and then shaped into small cakes. These were cooked in a stone baking pit that had been pre-heated through a series of fires and rakings of hot coals. Layers of leaves were placed in the hot oven and alternated with layers of the pine cakes. When the oven had been filled, the batch of cakes was covered with leaves and then topped with a mound of dry earth. After baking for an hour, the cakes were removed and smoked on a wooden frame over a cedar fire. The resulting bread was tough and black, but highly desired in times of scarcity. In this dried state pine-bark bread could be stored for months. Just prior to eating it was softened by boiling in water.

The following members of the great pine family were eaten in a variety of ways by some North American Indians.

ARBORVITAE

Although travelers through Canadian forests sometimes think of *The Maine Woods*, in which Thoreau chants "A quart of arbor-vitae, To make him strong and mighty," many remember that he rejected this tea of the twigs and wood chips as being too medicinal. Arborvitae, or White Cedar as it is sometimes called, is still utilized by some mountaineers for this tea which they insist is a valid cure for rheumatism. The Indians never mentioned this tea, but some ate the inner bark, or cambium, in emergencies or in times of scarcity.

This member of the great family of pines has leaves that are like flattened scales which overlap. The cones grow upright and are about one-half inch long. Arborvitae grows from eastern Quebec to Manitoba, south into the northeastern United States, and along the eastern mountains to Tennessee.

DOUGLAS FIR

The leaves of the Douglas fir have a very pleasant balsamic odor and were used when fresh as a substitute for coffee. This drink was a special favorite of the Yukis of California. The young twigs were sometimes boiled to make a refreshing drink by the Indians of British Columbia. As with the other conifers, the cambium layer was utilized as an emergency food.

Only the redwoods exceed this tree in height on the Pacific Coast. The Douglas fir grows over two hundred feet in height with a trunk diameter of two and a half to eight feet. The needles are flat and sharply pointed and about one inch long. The bark of the young Douglas fir is smooth and deeply fissured; on older trees it is reddish brown. The tree is relatively safe in fires, having a bark thickness of up to one foot. The cones hang downward and ripen in the fall when they drop to the forest floor. They are two to three inches long and have three-pronged bracts which are clearly visible, thus making this an easily identifiable species. Unfortunately, the Douglas fir is a favorite Christmas tree, and each year millions are cut from the forests of the Northwest.

❧ GRAND FIR

The Indians of British Columbia ate the inner bark of the grand fir in the spring when it was rich and juicy. To obtain this inner layer, or cambium, they separated the outer bark of the tree by using a sharpened piece of wood or a knife fashioned from an animal horn. The gummy "sap" of this and other firs was chewed as a gum and the juice swallowed for the nutrient contained.

This tall conifer pine grows straight and some-

times attains a height of one hundred and twenty-five feet. It has flat needles between one and one-fourth and two inches long, which grow opposite each other on the twigs. The needles are dark green and centrally grooved above, and silver to white below. Young trees have thin, even bark with many blisters, which exude a healing resin. Older trees are ridged. The cones are very apparent in late summer. They grow upright, are about one inch thick, and are between two and four inches long.

The grand fir is found in the northwestern United States and southwestern Canada, generally below three thousand feet in elevation.

❧ HEMLOCK (FIG. 128)

The various hemlocks were utilized throughout their range by groups of Indians who first

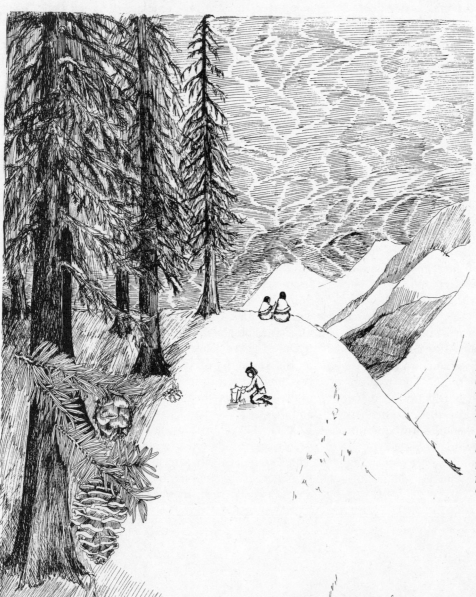

(FIG. 128) HEMLOCK: In the East, the young leaves of Canada hemlock were boiled into a drink by the Iroquois, while in the West the inner bark and sap of the western hemlock were dried and pressed into cakes or prepared like dough as bread.

discovered their nutritional value. In the East the young leaves of the Canada hemlock were boiled into a drink by the Iroquois. The inner bark and sap of the western hemlock were dried and pressed into cakes or prepared as a bread in Montana and British Columbia.

These trees grow between one hundred and twenty and one hundred and seventy-five feet high and have a characteristic droop on the topmost tip, which makes them easily identifiable from a distance. The long branches are spaced irregularly on the trunk and bear flat, blunt, dark green needles that grow densely around the twigs. The small cones grow downward, ripen in the fall, and drop during the winter. The tannin-rich bark is widely used in tanning, and the wood is in wide demand in the lumber industry. Hemlocks favor deep shade and are widely planted as ornamentals in Britain.

∾§ JUNIPER

The junipers make an excellent survival food because the berries, though somewhat bitter, are edible and available through part of the winter. Also, the inner bark is edible and was eaten by many Indians to fight off starvation. Some tribes preserved the berries by drying, then utilized them throughout the winter by baking these ground fruits into cakes or mush. Some Indian groups roasted juniper berries, ground them, and then used them as a coffee substitute. The Indians of British Columbia prepared an astringent tea by boiling the stems and leaves. New Mexican Indians used the berries from cherrystone juniper to flavor meats; they are said to impart a taste similar to sage. Juniper berries are used commercially to impart a flavor to gin.

Rocky Mountain juniper is prevalent in the western United States, south to New Mexico, and ranges from British Columbia to Alberta in Canada. It is generally a bushy shrub or small tree with several short trunks. The leaves are scalelike on older branches and needlelike on young shoots. The reddish brown bark is thin and stringy. Juniper berries are blue and are surrounded with a thin layer of fragrant wax that is easily removed by boiling.

∾§ LARCH

The Indians of British Columbia chewed the gummy exudate of the trunk and branches of the western larch for pleasure. Aside from the Ojibwa tribe, who drank a tea made of the roots of American larch, there are few Indian groups who relied on the larches as a source of food. The inner bark is probably edible and in Siberia the natives make a broth of this layer from a related species. The new shoots have been eaten by woodsmen in emergencies.

The western larch is easily recognized in the fall when it is yellow gold in color. Some varieties of this species grow up to eighty feet in height, while other varieties grow upwards of one hundred and sixty feet. These pines are irregular in form; their topmost limbs curve upwards, while the lower limbs generally twist downwards. The larches are important commercially since their heavy wood is in high demand for shoring and for other construction work.

∾§ PINES

Nearly all pine seeds are edible. The inner bark of the pine provides a nutritious emergency food that various tribes ate either raw or prepared and boiled. Some Indian groups dried the inner bark and stored it for later use. Below are listed some of the species of pine that were used as food by the American Indians.

∾§ DIGGER PINE

The digger pine, a well-known species, was an important food source for the Indians of California. The large cones contain sweet, oily nuts, which were favorites of the Digger Indians. These nuts are 28 percent protein and 51 percent fatty oil and were of great dietary importance in times of scarcity. To obtain the nuts, the Indians removed the resinous pitch from the cones and then tossed them into a fire to open the cone scales. The nuts were then beaten out. The Numlakis even held a ceremonial dance to celebrate the pine-nut season.

In addition to the above nutritive uses, the gum of the digger pine was highly prized for

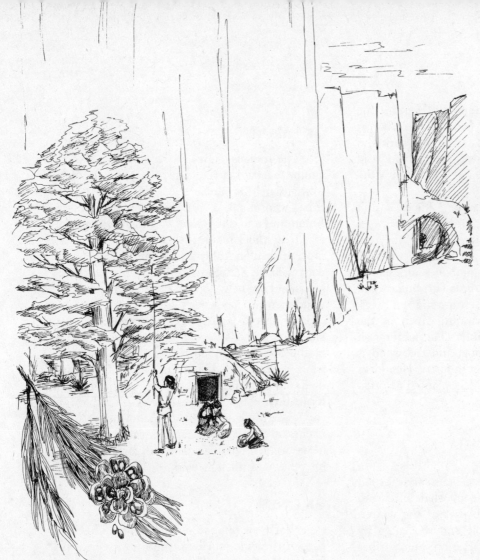

(FIG. 129) PIÑON: *The nuts of this pine tree were one of the choicest items in the Zuñi diet. They contain about 15 percent protein and were often ground into meal and used to make cakes.*

chewing. Older Indians chewed this gum to alleviate rheumatic pains, and the pitchy exudate was extensively applied to burns and cuts.

✎ PIÑON (FIG.129)

The nuts from the piñon species were at one time highly prized by southwestern tribes. They were one of the choicest items of the Zuñi diet. Piñon nuts were generally gathered after they had fallen from the trees, although in times of scarcity the branches were shaken to bring them down. These seeds are pleasant to the taste and fairly nutritious. They are about 15 percent protein, 62 percent oil, and 17 percent of other carbohydrates. The nuts were eaten raw; they were sometimes lightly toasted to improve the flavor or to dry them for storage. The seeds, with their coats removed, were ground into a meal and used to make cakes or to thicken soups. Some tribes mixed piñon nut meal with yucca seeds; others combined it with corn meal or sunflower seeds.

As with all pines, the needles make an invigorating outdoors tea when fresh, and the inner bark, though leathery, is edible.

✎ PONDEROSA PINE

The California tribes favored the digger pine and considered the nuts of the ponderosa pine too small for use as food, but Indians of the more interior regions of Montana, Idaho, Oregon, and British Columbia ate them raw and crushed them into a meal which was made into bread. These tribes also ate the mucilagenous inner bark and chewed the gummy exudate.

The roundish, light brown cones were used to make a quick fire, and the scales from the trunk bark burn easily, give off no smoke, and cool quickly. These bark scales were used for fires when Indian warriors wanted to conceal their movements.

The ponderosa is easily recognized by its orange red bark and the sheafs of three long needles.

✑ WHITE PINE

The Indians of New England boiled the needles of the white pine in water and drank the resulting tea to prevent scurvy. These needles contain up to five times as much vitamin C as is contained in an equal weight of lemons. White pine needles are also rich in vitamin A. The seeds were used to flavor meat in cooking by the Ojibwa. The sweet inner bark was frequently eaten by the Iroquois of New York State.

The early settlers of Massachusetts were quick to recognize the value of white pine; they valued this species so highly that all silver shillings struck in the late seventeenth century bore the image of this tree.

✑ SPRUCE

The Indians of Canada and the northern United States ate the inner bark of the spruce in a similar manner as they did the pines. Some tribes sucked on small spruce cones as a treat. The young shoots, stripped of the short needles, have also served as food in emergencies. All varieties of spruce were used as described above, but the black spruce, as described in "Earth Medicine," was used to save an early crew of explorers from scurvy. The bright green needles were boiled and the decoction drunk.

The black spruce grows across Canada, from the Pacific to the Atlantic Ocean, and for this reason it should be easily recognized by all nature lovers.

These trees generally have straight trunks and grow to a maximum height of fifty feet. The branches clump or bulge at the top, which make the tree easy to identify. The short, stiff needles are only one-half inch long, and the dark gray bark is very scaly. The round cones are small, grow in clusters, and often remain attached to the branches for years. At one time, great quantities of spruce beer were made from the young shoots.

THE ROSE AND GOOSEBERRY FAMILIES

Fruits and berries were eaten throughout North America as a regular part of the everyday diet of the Indian. They are the most conspicuous part of a food plant and often the most delicious in the raw state. Although they do not contain great bulk, these small fruits contain much water and are generally high in the essential vitamins. It is not possible nor relevant to list all of the fleshy fruits and berries that formed a part of the Indian diet, but several preparations will be described. The simplest rule to follow regarding the use of wild fruits is to learn the poisonous species of your region since they comprise a very small minority in relation to the total number of edible varieties.

In the West, those berries which were most widely eaten were the bearberry, blackberry, blueberry, bullberry, chokeberry, currant, elderberry, hawthorn, raspberry, serviceberry, and the thimbleberry. Although most of these fruits were eaten in the fresh state or preserved by drying, the thimbleberry was eaten raw and never dried for storage among the Indians of Mendocino County. A root tea of the common blackberry of that region was commonly used to arrest diarrhea.

In the East, the principal berries used by the Iroquois were the blackberry, blueberry, currant, cranberry, dewberry, elderberry, gooseberry, huckleberry, mulberry, partridgeberry, raspberry, serviceberry (Juneberry), strawberry, sumacberry, thimbleberry, and the wintergreen.

These berries were gathered in season by the women and eaten raw, crushed with maple sugar and water, or added to puddings. For use during the winter, certain of these fruits were dried by exposure to the sun, namely, the blackberry, blueberry, huckleberry, and the black raspberry. When removed from storage, the dried berries were soaked in water and slowly heated with maple sugar added. The Iroquois ate these preserved berries as described or mixed them with bread meal or hominy.

The anthropologist of Iroquois origin, A. C. Parker, describes the fun of berrying among his people:

The gathering of the autumn berries was regarded more of a pastime than work. In fact, work with these people in many lines was made easier by its social character, and seemed more like a game where the thrill of it all kept the thought of fatigue away. . . . The women and girls . . . would go in groups to the places where patches of the vines and bushes grew and sing their folksongs as they gathered the fruit. Everyone laughed or sang and picked as fast as their two hands could touch the berries.

As the berries filled the baskets they were protected from the heat of the sun by sumac or basswood leaves. Parker continues, describing an interesting snake repellent:

In picking mountain huckleberries or those which grew in snake infested places the moccasins were smeared with lard to frighten away the rattlers. The snakes, scenting the hog fat, would think that pigs were scouting for them.

Indian tribes throughout North America commonly made cakes of the small, fleshy berries of their region. The fruits were first pounded and then boiled by the addition of hot stones to a bark vessel filled with water. After boiling, the berries were placed on pine needles or other leaves in thick masses and allowed to dry. As they dried and formed cakes, the juice which had been removed from them during the boiling was poured back into the "batter." These flavorful cakes were mainly used in stews and puddings but were also eaten by themselves.

Berries were sometimes mixed with dried meat that had been pulverized to a powder. Boiled, melted animal fat was added to the mixture, the dried mass forming the famous pemmican, an important Indian survival food. Since this solid food was readily carried on long journeys, it was adopted by the early settlers and soon formed an important part of their wilderness food supply.

Some of the fruits which were eaten by the Indian include the following.

✑ CHERRIES

Black cherries were eaten fresh or dried for future use. They were pulverized in a stone mortar and combined with dried, powdered meat and added to soups. Some tribes enjoyed a tea of the twigs as an invigorating beverage. Although the chokeberry was never considered a delicious variety, certain northern tribes dried and pounded them, removed the bitter acid from the "pits," and baked the mass as pemmican. The pin cherry was eaten raw and was quickly adopted by the settlers, who learned to recognize this early appearing, light red fruit. The sand cherry, which grows on sand bars and along the banks of rivers in the northeastern states, produces the largest of our native cherries, often up to half an inch across. These red fruits are slightly bitter but were eaten fresh or preserved by the Indians.

✑ CRAB APPLE

The native crab apples occur throughout most of the United States and were generally too tart to be eaten in the raw state. The Indians gathered them in the fall and stored them in bark containers in the ground. In the springtime, the fruits were sweet to the taste and were made into jelly, syrup, or cider.

The Iroquois were especially fond of the apple,

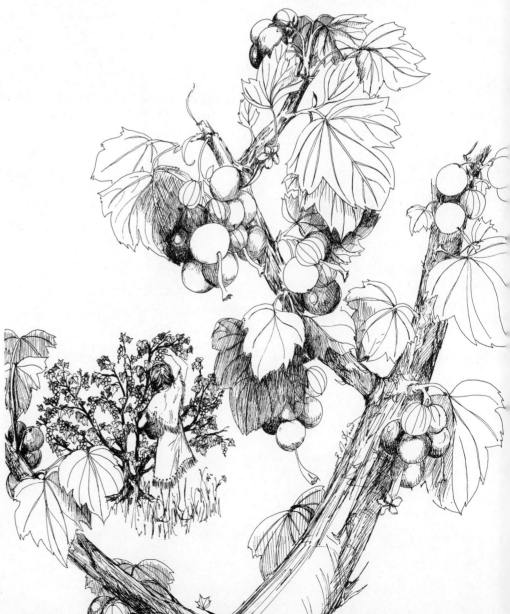

(FIG. 130) CURRANT: Many native varieties of currant were eaten by the Indians. Some tribes boiled the young leaves and ate them with uncooked animal fat.

preferring the true apples, which they ate raw, as sauce, or baked in the hot embers of a campfire. For drying, apples were strung from poles or hung over the stove on twine.

CURRANT (FIG.130)

More than thirteen edible varieties of currant occur in North America, and all were eaten either fresh or dried by the Indian. Some tribes boiled the young leaves in early spring and ate them with uncooked animal fat. Several wilderness recipes recommend the honey-rich flowers as food, adding that the Indians cautioned against consuming too much of the fruit.

During World War II, as a result of the shortage of oranges, black currants were grown in England for their high vitamin C content and used in children's and infants' foods.

GOOSEBERRY

Many wild varieties of gooseberry were eaten fresh, cooked, or preserved by the Indian. To remove the bristly spines which are found on some species, the berries were rolled on hot coals in baskets until the spines had been singed off.

WILD ROSE

The Indian did not suffer from scurvy, probably because he ate so many vitamin-C-rich berries throughout the year. Varieties of the wild rose were eaten from British Columbia to Maine, and it has been determined that their seed pods or hips contain large quantities of this important vitamin. Three rose hips are said to contain as much vitamin C as one orange.

During World War II the English people were encouraged to gather the red fruits left on hedges following the blooming period of the wild rose. These were pulverized and distributed by the Ministry of Health throughout the country for their important vitamin content.

The Indians generally ate these fruits in the raw state in times of scarcity. They are available throughout the year, are easily recognized, and probably should be sought out by all those interested in natural foods of high nutritional value. In addition to containing up to sixty times as much vitamin C as lemons, rose hips are richer in calcium, phosphorus, and iron than oranges. This is hardly a native food to be overlooked.

SEAWEEDS, MUSHROOMS, AND LICHENS

The seaweeds were a minor food of the Indians and were eaten mainly by tribes of the Pacific Coast, north to Alaska. Laver (FIG.131) was commonly eaten fresh or baked. These red algae are very pleasant tasting and are consumed

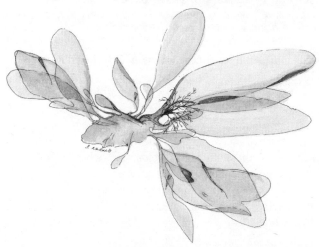

(FIG. 131) LAVER: *These red algae comprise most of the world's edible seaweed and were eaten by tribes of the Pacific Coast.*

in large quantities by the Japanese and Chinese. Certain Asian varieties, known as *nori*, comprise most of the world's edible seaweed; their cultivation comprises a major marine agricultural industry.

The red seaweeds are best gathered from the end of winter through summer, when they are thickest and best for eating.

ᴥ KELP (EDIBLE) (FIG.132)

This broad "leaved" algae grows in large beds in Alaskan waters and along the northeastern coast of the United States. Tribes in both regions first removed the broad membrane, then ate the thick midrib for its sweet flavor. As is true with most seaweeds, edible kelp is rich in iodine and

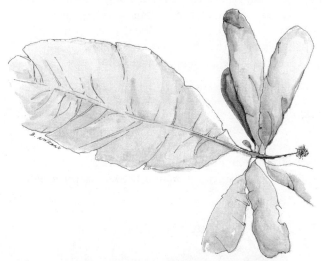

(FIG. 132) KELP: *This broad-leaved seaweed was eaten by tribes in Alaska and along the northeastern coast. The broad membrane was first removed and the thick midrib eaten for its sweet flavor.*

may have served to prevent goiter among the Indians who ate it.

As Western man runs short of cultivated land plants, he too may turn to the seaweeds for survival.

New interest in the algae has even yielded a promising drug possibility. Although the primitive Hawaiians were a large and fat people, they had no known heart disease. Researchers are now investigating a seaweed which was eaten as a flavoring, *limu lipoa*. This seaweed degrades fats to a highly unsaturated oil and may have been partially responsible for the low incidence of coronary occlusions.

Many edible varieties of mushrooms were eaten raw or cooked and added to other foods, soups, etc. Since many fungi are deadly, only a few of the edible species will be listed. The interested reader is directed to other books which are devoted solely to these tricky plants. As a general rule, the beginner should avoid all wild mushrooms until he learns the characteristics of all poisonous species. Some of the more easily recognized fungi which were eaten by the Indians are listed below.

✍§ ELM CAP

Indians of the Dakota Nation gathered elm caps—long, thick mushrooms—from decayed areas of elms or box elders. This mushroom is particularly abundant after heavy rains and is not limited to elm trees.

✍§ MEADOW MUSHROOM (FIG.133)

These short, white to brown mushrooms were relished by the Iroquois who boiled them after peeling and dicing. The meadow mushroom is the most common mushroom of the market

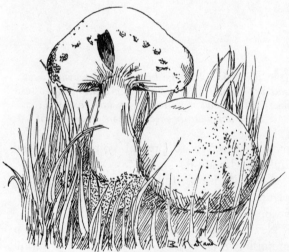

(FIG. 133) MEADOW MUSHROOM: *This common mushroom of the marketplace was relished by the Iroquois, who boiled it after peeling and dicing, just as we do today.*

place, and is found growing wild in pastures, on lawns, along roadsides, etc. They are most delicious when gathered from late summer through early fall.

✍§ PUFFBALLS (FIG.134)

The round to balloon-shaped puffballs were eaten in their early stages of growth, either raw, boiled, or roasted. The Zuñis dried them for

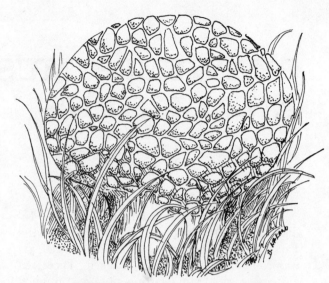

(FIG. 134) PUFFBALLS: *These round- to balloon-shaped mushrooms were eaten in their early stages of growth either raw, boiled, or roasted.*

winter use, while the Iroquois fried them and added them to soups.

Various species of puffballs are edible and all are harmless when young. They have white flesh and discolored individuals must be rejected. The giant puffball may grow to more than one foot in diameter and is found in fields and rich woods. It is the largest edible fungus and is easily recognized by its round shape. The Omaha Indians cut this large, delicious species into chunks and fried it like meat.

✍§ BRACKET FUNGI

Bracket fungi, sulphur yellow to orange brackets which grow on the bases of decayed or dead trees, were sliced and then boiled for more than thirty minutes before they were eaten. The Dakota Indians ate only the young ones and avoided those found on ash trees, owing to their bitterness. The Hopi avoided all brackets because they associated them with the malignant growths of cancer and feared contamination.

✍§ SMUTS

Several tribes gathered smuts as they appeared on corn plants and boiled them as a food. The Hopis enjoyed this food, too, but they held that "smut found on a man's corn is considered a sign that he has defecated in his field. . . ."

Although the lichens were not regarded as common foods, in emergencies many types were eaten. They were scraped from rocks or trees and eaten raw or boiled with fat. To remove the bitter taste, some tribes washed them in water mixed with the ashes of a campfire.

Lichens belong to a large plant group and are found in diverse habitats on every continent. They survive under extreme conditions of heat and cold, and in these environments, man has learned to live on them in the absence of other foods.

One of the most obvious species is the reindeer moss (FIG.135), which covers great areas of northern Canada. Reindeer and caribou depend on this carpet of food for survival, and in this sense, among the northern tribes, an entire food chain begins with this one species. When eaten by man it is either boiled as a soup or dried, powdered, and baked as bread.

Two other species of edible lichens are Iceland moss and rock tripe. Both abound in the northern regions and were usually boiled to a nutritious and palatable jelly before they were eaten.

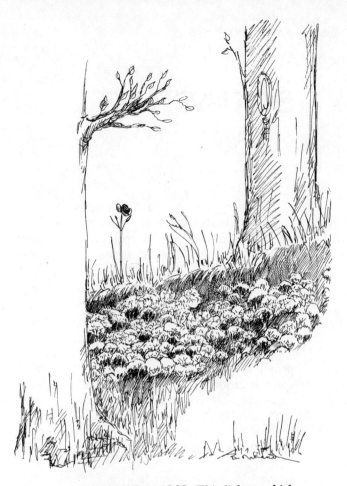

(FIG. 135) REINDEER MOSS: *This lichen, which covers great areas of northern Canada, makes an excellent survival food. When prepared for human consumption it is either boiled as a soup or dried, powdered, and baked as bread.*

SQUASHES

The Iroquois cultivated cucumbers, cantaloupes, and watermelons in woods that had been cleared by fire for that purpose. Before winter they gathered the vines of those melons which had not yet ripened, leaving the roots undisturbed. These melons were stored in baskets of sand and kept in lodges during the winter. As they ripened, they were given to the sickest members of the tribe.

Although the Iroquois were a great communal people they recognized individual rights with respect to melons, as we learn from A. C. Parker:

Those who planted melons in cleared woodland tracts set up poles upon which were painted the clan totems and the name signs of the owners.

The totem sign signified that while, according to the communistic laws, the patch belonged, nominally, to the clan, and that any clansman might take the fruit if necessary, yet by virtue of the fact that the garden was cleared, planted and cultivated by the individual whose name was indicated, the individual claim and right should be recognized as actually prior, though not nominally.

The squashes (FIG.136) contained some of the most important foods of the Indian diet as described below.

✌ CANTALOUPES

Cantaloupes may have been introduced to the New World by Columbus in 1494. Cartier

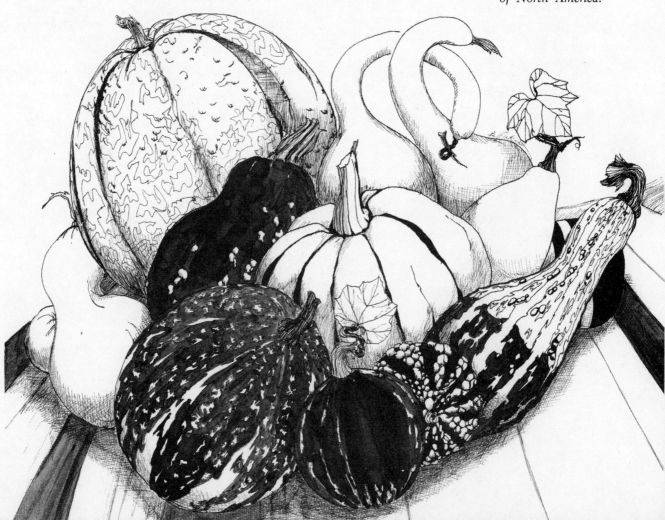

(FIG. 136) *Some GOURD Varieties Eaten by the Indians of North America.*

found these melons under cultivation at Hoche-laga (now Montreal) during his second voyage to North America, and by 1881 cantaloupes which had been grown in Montreal were being sold in Boston.

⋘ CUCUMBERS

Cucumbers have been cultivated since ancient times and are thought to have originated in western Asia. This vegetable was cultivated by several Indian tribes. Cartier, the French explorer, reported that as early as 1535 the Indians of the present site of Montreal cultivated "very great cucumbers."

⋘ PUMPKINS AND SQUASHES

Next to corn, pumpkins and squashes were probably the most important cultivated plants. In addition to supplying the Indian with a highly nutritious food, many utensils (water bottles, dishes, etc.), religious objects (masks), and musical instruments (rattles, horns, flutes) were made from them. They averaged about 10 percent protein by weight, while the buffalo-gourd contained up to 23 percent protein.

The Iroquois preserved these vegetables by cutting them into thin pieces and suspending the dried sections on cord from the ceilings of their lodges. Squashes were simply baked in the hot embers of a fire and then eaten, the shell and seeds included. Sometimes squashes were cleaned of seeds and then boiled in water. In the Southwest, the Navajo prepared squash in several ways. The vegetables were cut in quarters and roasted in stone ovens, in hot embers, or on open flames. They were sometimes sliced into small pieces, boiled in water, and salted, or fried in sheep fat. For storage purposes squashes were thoroughly dried in strips and parched over hot embers.

The Iroquois boiled infertile squash flowers with other foods as a special flavoring, while the Navajo boiled them with lamb fat as a soup. Squash blossoms were often gathered when they were big, dried in the shade on cord, and stored for use during the winter when they were used to flavor soups and meats.

Sturtevant includes the words of an early Dutch visitor to this country who described his impressions of the pumpkin around 1642:

The natives have another species of this vegetable peculiar to themselves. . . . the plant was not known to us before our intercourse with them. It is a delightful fruit, as well to the eye on account of its fine variety of colors, as to the mouth for its agreeable taste. . . . It is gathered in summer, and when it is planted in the middle of April, the fruit is fit for eating by the first of June. They do not wait for it to ripen before making use of the fruit, but only until it has attained a certain size.

⋘ WATERMELONS

Watermelons were cultivated by tribes in Arizona, North and South Dakota, Minnesota, Nebraska, New York, and Wisconsin. The watermelon originated in tropical Africa and appears to have been introduced to America by European colonists as early as the seventeenth century. The first watermelons in Connecticut were grown from seeds that had been transported from Russia. By 1822 large melons were reported growing in Illinois. Writes one J. Woods:

Watermelons are also in great plenty, of vast size; some I suppose weigh 20 pounds. They are more like pumpkins in outward appearance than melons. They are round or oblong, generally green, or a green and whitish color on the outside, and white or pale on the inside, with many black seeds in them, very juicy, in flavor like rich water, and sweet and mawkish, but cool and pleasant.

At least one scientist, M. R. Gilmore, traced the varieties of watermelons found in North America and concluded that many of them were native to this continent and were grown here long before the introduction of the European varieties.

Among the Hopi, the watermelon was sometimes a staple food. These Indians regretted having traded their "old type" melons which kept until February for newer varieties which were better flavored, but which did not keep as well, as they related to the ethnobotanist A. F. Whiting in the 1930s.

MISCELLANEOUS

In this large section I have included many useful plants which do not belong to any of the families already described. Although some important Indian food plants do not appear here, such as the skunk cabbage or the Indian turnip, they are described elsewhere in this book under medicines.

The first three plants, the arrowhead, the cattail, and the water lily, all occur in marshes, ponds, lakes, and streams throughout North America and are grouped together. All the other miscellaneous food plants are arranged alphabetically.

ARROWHEAD (WAPATOO)
(FIG.137,c)

Long before the arrival of the European, the Wapatoo was traded between tribes in local commerce, especially among the Chinooks of Oregon, where the tubers were a chief article of food. As Lewis and Clark reported, "this bulb forms a principal article of traffic between the inhabitants of the Vally and those of their neighbourhood or sea coast."

The Indian method of gathering these bulbs was unique. The women entered the water, sometimes up to their necks, supported themselves by hanging on to a canoe, and rooted out the tubers with their toes. The loosened bulbs immediately rose to the surface of the water and were gathered. It is not possible to secure these tubers by pulling the plant from the water, as they break off readily and remain lodged in the muddy bottom.

The smooth tubers were occasionally eaten raw, but more frequently they were roasted like potatoes and served with other foods.

The arrowhead grows in the mud of shallow waters throughout most of the United States. The arrow-shaped leaves are easily recognized, and the white flowers appear in whorls of three. As an emergency food it is readily available throughout the year.

CATTAIL (FIG.137,a)

The cattails grow throughout North America and were highly regarded as food plants by the Indians. Various tribes reported that they cut the young shoots from the roots in the spring, peeled off the leaves, and ate the succulent interior portion fresh. The Paiutes ate the young flower stalks—before the pollen was produced—either fresh or boiled. The flowers themselves were eaten alone or in soups, breads, or puddings. The pollen makes excellent flour and was baked into bread, etc. The young rootstocks are also edible, and the Indians ate the white interior after removing the outer layer. These new rootstocks are recognized by the buds which appear at their ends, the sign of new growth about to begin. Another use for the starchy rootstocks is as flour. After drying, they are readily pulverized between stones, the fibers removed, and the flour is ready for baking. Finally, the down was removed from the spikes, charred, and the seeds eaten. (Cattail down was also used as padding in bedding and pillows and as diapers prior to the introduction of cotton fabrics.)

WATER LILY (POND LILY)
(FIG.137,b)

In the Northwest the Klamath Indians regarded the time of ripening of their native yellow pond lily with a religious fervor. Ceremonial dances were held before all tribe members participated in harvesting the ripe seeds. The large pods were dried in the sun and then pounded to loosen the seeds. The seeds were then slightly parched on hot stones and pounded to separate the useful kernels from the shells. The kernels were either ground into flour or roasted and eaten or stored for future use. The rootstocks, too, were eaten, but they had to be gathered from the muddy bottoms of the lakes, ponds, or streams in which they are found. These thick rootstocks were rarely eaten raw; they were usually boiled or

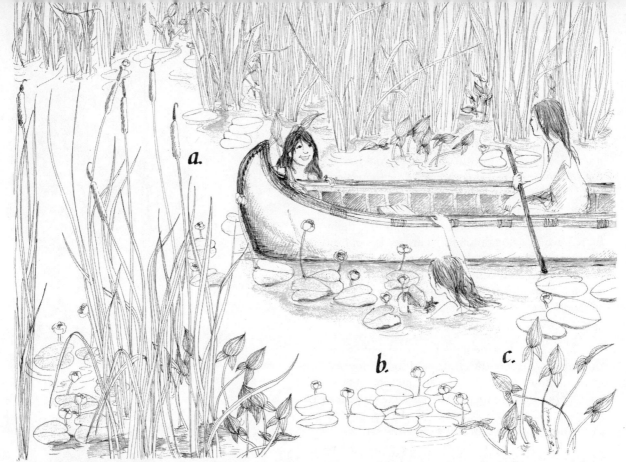

(FIG. 137) *Some Native Food Plants Found in Marshes, Ponds, and Lakes: (a)* CATTAIL *(left); (b)* WATER LILY *(center); (c)* ARROWHEAD *(lower right).*

baked and their rinds removed before the sweet centers were eaten. Of course, the starchy root-stocks were also ground into flour and used for making bread or thin porridge.

The yellow pond lily which is commonly found east of the Rocky Mountains was eaten by Indians of Montana, the Dakotas, Wisconsin, and the northeastern states. The roots were gathered by the women in a similar manner to the gathering of arrowhead—namely, by using the toes. These tuberous roots were also stolen from muskrat dens, but only when the animals themselves were hunted. The Iroquois believed it would be dangerous to invite the vengeance of these animals by stealing their food and leaving them hungry.

Women of the Plains tribes also took food from the burrows of animals, but they went so far as to leave some other edible food in place of that which they "borrowed." As women of the Dakota Nation gathered stores of beans from muskrat dens, left equal quantities of corn, an abundant food item. Gilmore, the ethnologist, reports: "They said it would be wicked to steal from the animals, but they thought that a fair exchange was not robbery." This, no doubt, was done out of concern for the animal spirits, but the food exchange certainly assured survival of the useful ground dwellers.

The eastern species was prepared exactly as the western pond lily; the rootstocks were boiled or roasted or used for flour, while the seeds were parched and eaten or ground into flour.

The water chinquapin also grows in a water environment and was an important food of the Indians. The long rootstocks bear extensions which were gathered during the fall for their starchy pulp, and the hard seeds were eaten after their shells were removed or cooked with meat. The plant has large air spaces throughout. This anatomical rarity brought some of the Plains tribes to believe that anyone who dug the tubers must not "snuffle" through his nostrils for fear that the air cavities of the plants would be filled with mud and spoiled!

This plant is nearly extinct and is not detailed for that reason. Nevertheless, should the reader find himself in an emergency situation and be fortunate enough to locate the largest water lily of the northeastern United States, he could easily proceed to gather the tubers as he would with the tuberous roots of the arrowhead or the yellow pond lily; he could eat the seeds, either in the unripe state when they are delicious raw, or in the ripe stage after crushing and winnowing them to remove the tough shells. The seeds contain up to 19 percent protein, are available throughout the year (especially during summer and fall), and make an excellent emergency food.

✑ AGAVE (FIG.138)

The several varieties of agave that grow throughout the Southwest to California formed an important part of the economy of several tribes. One Indian group, the Mescalero Apaches, received their name because of the fermented drink *mescal* which they made from the sap. They simply bored into the middle of the plant at the base of the long flower stalk, tapped the sap into a container, and after fermenting it, distilled it into their favorite drink (which was also called *pulque*).

Several tribes used the bud which appears at the base of the flower stalk for food. These were sometimes as large as two feet across. They were slowly baked in large stone–earth ovens for several days. This nutritious, fibrous product tasted sweet and is said to be a useful scurvy preventative. The baked plant bud was sometimes dried after baking, pounded into flat sheets, and stored for times of need. Among the Apaches this was a staple article of food.

A species of agave which is common in Mexico, century plant, was so useful that the historian Prescott called it the "miracle of nature." From the leaves the Aztecs made a paper which resembled papyrus. Twine was manufactured from the tough leaf fibers. The gelatinous pulp was used with water to produce a frothy soaplike lather. Waterproof roofing was secured from the dried flower stalks, and the leaf thorns were used for needles. A black dye was made from the top of the flower stalk and used in ceremonial body painting.

The most common agave of the Mojave Desert (*A. utahensis*) is easily recognized, especially in its flowering period. From late spring through

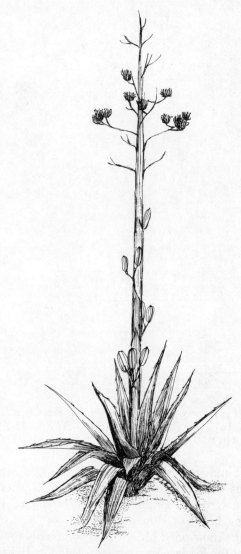

(FIG. 138) AGAVE: *Varieties of the agave were used throughout the Southwest as food, in the preparation of a fermented drink, for twine, to make soap, in the construction of shelters, etc.*

July yellow blossoms appear on its rapidly ascending central stalk. The plant blooms just once and then dies.

Agave may be mistaken for datil yucca, but it should be easy to distinguish by the spines which appear on the margins of its leaves and by the ovaries which grow *beneath* its flowers.

All species of agave can be used in emergencies, the bud needing only to be roasted in the hot embers of a good fire.

✑ AMARANTH (FIG.139)

Amaranth resembles the lamb's-quarters or pigweeds and is scattered throughout North

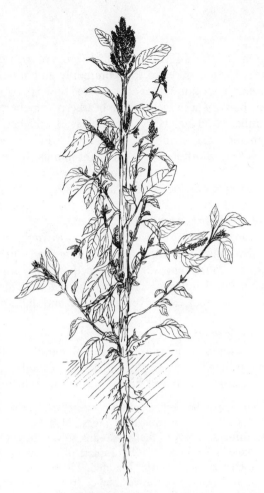

(FIG. 139) AMARANTH: *The Indians of Arizona cultivated these plants for their small black seeds. The seeds were parched and eaten whole or ground into flour.*

The wild plants have thickened roots which are edible, but which are too small to consider as a food staple. Nevertheless, the roots, after boiling, would be good in emergencies. They re-

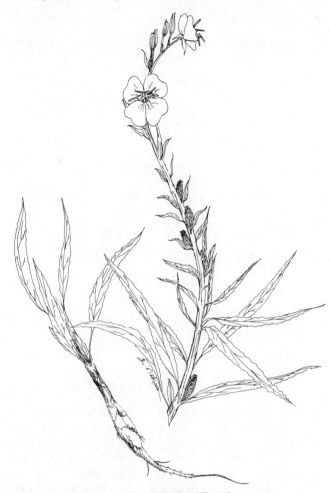

(FIG. 140) EVENING PRIMROSE: *The young stems and leaves of almost all varieties of this plant have been used as food. The roots are tough and small but can, after boiling, be eaten in an emergency.*

America as a weed. Nevertheless, it produces many small, black seeds which were so highly valued by the Indians of Arizona that they cultivated them. The seeds were parched and eaten whole or ground into flour.

The leaves and stems of young plants were used for greens by the Indians and then by the early settlers and are said to make an excellent spinach when cooked.

EVENING PRIMROSE (FIG.140)

Certain varieties of the evening primrose (*O. albicaulis, O. brevipes*) have seed pods and were eaten by the Indians. Almost all varieties have been eaten for their young stems and leaves, and as early as 1614 it was introduced to Europe, where it was soon cultivated for its edible leaves, shoots, and roots.

portedly taste best when gathered in late fall, winter, and early spring.

By day, these plants appear as wilted individuals, but at dusk the larger buds open quickly and bear large, beautiful flowers with soft, silky petals.

FIREWEED (FIG.141)

Fireweed is often one of the earliest to appear in areas that have been burned out. In British Columbia, the Indians peel the stalks and eat the

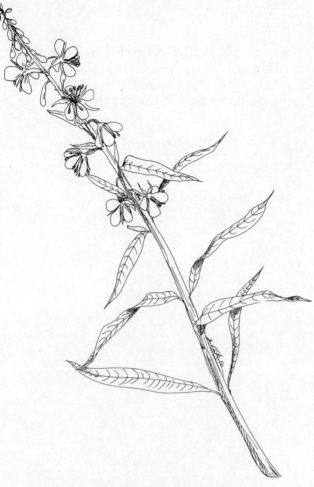

(FIG. 141) FIREWEED: *This plant is one of the earliest to appear in areas that have been burned out. In British Columbia, the Indians peel the stalks and eat the pith fresh or cook it as soup.*

gelatinous pith fresh or cook it as soup. Some tribes use the core for breadmaking.

The young shoots are eaten by some campers who cook it like asparagus. The flower stalks and leaves are eaten in salads. For these purposes the fireweed was introduced to Europe, where it is still a popular vegetable in certain countries.

Fireweed is abundant in burned lands and literally thousands of acres of its magenta blossoms soothe the observer's image of fire-blackened areas. These plants make excellent vegetables and should be easy to recognize. In the Gaspe Peninsula, the French Canadians value it so that they call this herb *asperge*, or wild asparagus.

❧ MANZANITA (FIG.142)

The manzanita belongs to the heath family. In this group we find many plants which were eaten by the Indian but which are not treated here because they are still commonly and simply eaten, or because they are treated elsewhere in this book. These include the bearberry, blueberry, cranberry, dangleberry, deerberry, huckleberry, Labrador tea, madrone, pipsissewa, wintergreen, and the whortleberry. This plant family is well represented by several ornamental shrubs, namely, the laurels, rhododendrons, and the azaleas. From the food point of view, of course, the blueberries and cranberries are the best known.

Aside from eating their wild berries fresh, the Indians also sun-dried them and ground them into a "flour" that was later added as a flavoring to breads, soups, etc. The dried berries were also mixed with dried pulverized meat and fat and carried on long journeys.

An interesting recipe for making manzanita cider comes to us from the ethnobotanist V. K. Chestnut who visited the Indians of Round Valley, California, at the beginning of this century:

> The ripe berries, carefully selected to exclude those that are worm-eaten, are scalded for a few minutes, or until the seeds are soft, when the whole is crushed. . . . To a quart of this pulp an equal quantity of water is added. The mass is then poured immediately over some dry pine needles

(FIG. 142) MANZANITA: *The ripe berries of this bush were used by the Indians of Round Valley, California, to prepare a delicious cider.*

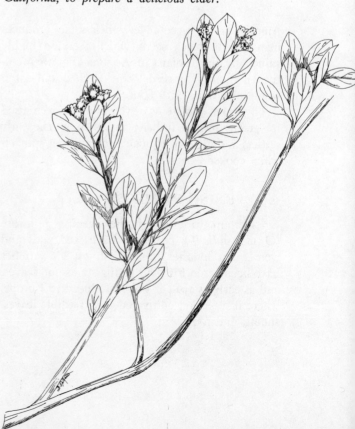

or straw contained in a shallow sieve basket, and the cider is allowed to drain into a water-tight basket placed beneath, or sometimes it is allowed to stand an hour or so and then strained. After cooling, the cider is ready for use. . . . It is delightfully spicy and acid in taste. . . . it seems probable that some of the Indians not only ferment the cider to obtain vinegar, but also to obtain an alcoholic beverage.

It should be noted that the same writer reported that several fatalities occurred from the overeating of manzanita berries:

Death is said to occur from eating the fruit too freely. The bowels become stopped with great masses of seeds and pulp and death follows, with contraction of the pupils and general tetanic spasms, such as one observed with strychnine poisoning or in the symptoms of cerebrospinal meningitis.

This observation is puzzling because other writers on the subject categorically list the fruits of various species of manzanita as edible without adding any note of caution.

⤚§ MINER'S LETTUCE (FIG.143,a)

Miner's lettuce, an easily recognized herb, saved many California gold miners from scurvy. Too busy in their search for gold, many of them neglected to plant vegetable gardens and looked to the wild plants for their much needed greens. Again the native American provided critical help to a mass of foreigners who eventually ran them off the lands of their ancestors.

Miner's lettuce is one of our most easily recognized native plants. It has two types of leaves. The lower ones are on long stalks, while its upper leaves are united and form a shroudlike arrangement through which the stem passes. It thrives in moist soil, on slopes, and occurs throughout the western United States.

Leslie L. Haskin, in his book on Pacific Coast flora, cites an interesting Indian recipe for these succulent leaves. It is taken from Stephen Powers, "Tribes of California":

The Indians living in the mountains gather it and lay it in quantities near the nests of certain large red ants, which have the habit of building conical heaps over their holes. After the ants have circulated all through it, they take it up, and shake

them off, and eat it with relish. They say the ants, in running over it, impart a sour taste to it, and make it as good as if it had vinegar on it.

Of course, it would be just as simple to add a little vinegar if you don't take well to this recipe. Another wild green that is rich in vitamin C is

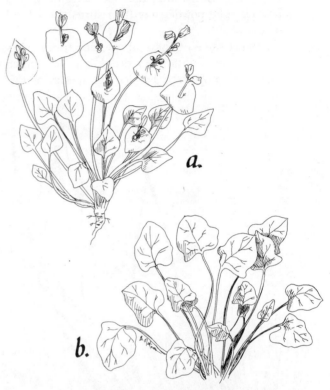

(FIG. 143) (a) MINER'S LETTUCE: This easily recognized herb saved many California gold miners from scurvy; (b) SCURVY GRASS: The bright green leaves of this northerly herb were collected and eaten in large quantities by European seamen to prevent scurvy.

scurvy grass (FIG.143,b). It grows in northern regions from Alaska to Newfoundland and was important to seamen of the early 1800s who were continually threatened by scurvy.

It is not known whether the Indians were aware of the usefulness of this plant; however, the bright green leaves were collected in large quantities and packed aboard ships in bales by the early European explorers. The plant has the strong odor of horseradish (to which it is related botanically) and is widely distributed in northern North America on seashores and sea cliffs. It belongs to the mustard family, as do cabbage, turnips, cauliflower, Brussels sprouts, watercress, etc.

MORMON TEA (FIG.144)

Mormon tea, a primitive-looking shrub which is common in the deserts and dry plains of the West, was used for making tea by both the Indians and the early pioneers. The green twigs were used, usually after they had been dried to a powder. The powder was then stirred in a bowl of warm water.

Among some of the southwestern tribes, Mormon tea was most often drunk for its reputed medicinal properties. The various species of this plant were widely used to cure venereal disease.

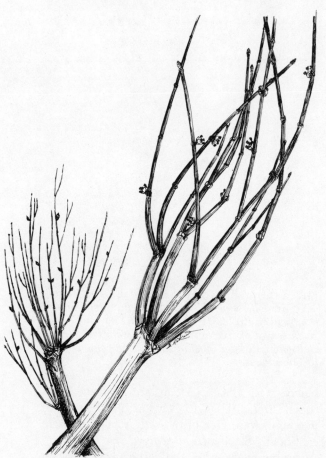

(FIG. 144) MORMON TEA: *The green twigs of these primitive-looking shrubs were used for tea both by the Indians and by the early pioneers.*

One Navajo remedy consisted of burning the plant with charcoal in a hole in the ground in the center of the hogan. The afflicted individual then squatted over the hole and allowed the black smudge to touch his diseased organ in the belief that this would effect a cure.

If Mormon tea had been drunk only for medicinal purposes it would have been best entered in the preceding section. This was not the case, however. Many people, especially the settlers and some Indians of this century, drank these teas solely as a pleasant-tasting beverage. Further, some tribes roasted the seeds and ground them into flour which was used in bread making, or ate them whole.

SPIDER LILY

Several tribes reportedly ate the leaves of the spider lily as greens after cooking or consumed the young shoots of this beautiful plant fresh. The ethnologist M. R. Gilmore described the poetic use of this graceful lily among some Plains tribes:

> When a young man of the Dakota Nation is in love, and walking alone on the prairie he finds this flower blooming, he sings to it a song in which he personifies it with the qualities of his sweetheart's character as they are called to his mind by the characteristics figuratively displayed by the flower before him. In his mind the beauties of the flower and of the girl are mutually transmitted and flow together into one image.

It seems beautiful that a plant that was used for food by one group of Indians was regarded with such poetic love by another; witness this Dakota song to the spider lily as it appears in Gilmore's work:

> Wee little dewy flower,
> So blessed and so shy,
> Thou'rt dear to me, and for
> My love for thee I'd die.

More than a native flora was plowed over on the plains.

EARTH FLAVORINGS

As the earth holds all the needs of man, so does man hold all the needs of earth. And in this common nurturance the great creator provides condiments and flavorings, garnishes and savories.

Any kind of food, no matter how nutritious, soon goes bland when eaten for several meals in succession. The "noble savage" also required his spices of life and found them in the mountains, on the plains, along the shores.

Salt, being *essential* as a preservative for meat

held over the lean winter months, was so important in the economies of Indian peoples that *wars* were fought—in California, at least—over access to beds of the crystal on Pacific shores.

Native wild mints were popular among the colonists when foreign spices and herb gardens failed. Necessity forced the European visitors to search for and enjoy the offerings long enjoyed by American natives.

TASTY MINTS

Latin Name	Common Name	Where and How Utilized
Agastache anethiodora	Giant hyssop	Leaf "tea" used in Nebraska, Wyoming, Montana, Dakotas
Agastache neomexicana		Leaves as food flavoring in New Mexico
Agastache urticifolia		Seeds eaten in Nevada and Utah
Hedeoma drummondii	Pennyroyal variety	Flowering tops infused as drink in Texas
Hedeoma nana	Pennyroyal variety	Leaves chewed for flavor in New Mexico
Koellia virginiana	Virginia mountain-mint	Flowers and buds for seasoning by Chippewas
Lycopus asper		Dried rootstocks boiled in Minnesota and Wisconsin
Lycopus virginicus		Rootstocks boiled as food in British Columbia
Mentha canadensis	American wild mint	Leaves infused as drink; eaten in Wisconsin, Montana, Wyoming, Utah, Oregon, Nevada, and Arizona

TASTY MINTS (continued)

Latin Name	Common Name	Where and How Utilized
Micromeria chamissonis		Leafy vines dried, used as tea substitute in California
Monarda citriodora	Lemon bee balm	Hopis boiled whole plant and ate it with hares
Monarda didyma	Oswego tea	Oswegos used leaves as tea substitute
Monarda fistulosa	Wild bergamot	Whole plant used in cooking meat in New Mexico
Monarda pectinata	Pony bee balm	Leaves used as seasoning in New Mexico
Monardella lanceolata		California tribes used whole plant as tea substitute
Monardella sheltonii		California tribes used leaves as tea substitute
Nepeta cataria	Catnip	Ojibwas utilized leaves as tea substitute
Pogogyne parviflora		California tribes used seeds as flavoring in pinole, leaves as tea substitute
Poliomintha incana		Arizona tribes boiled leaves or salted them raw as relish; used flowers as flavoring
Prunella vulgaris	Self-heal	British Columbians drank cold-water infusion of whole plant
Ramona incana		Southwestern natives made meal of ground seeds
Ramona polystachya	White bee-sage	California natives ate stem-tops and seeds
Ramona stachyoides		Seeds eaten in California
Salvia ballotaeflora		Texas natives made drink of flowering tops
Salvia carduacea	Thistle sage	California tribes roasted and ground seeds into meal; also used for a cooling drink

TASTY MINTS (continued)

Latin Name	Common Name	Where and How Utilized
Salvia columbariae	California chia	Seeds for drinks and soups, in Arizona and California
Stachys scopulorum		Seeds a food in Utah and Nevada

Plato recognized the need for wild greens as a "relish" in his *Republic*. Of course, such salad plants have been eaten by all peoples close to the earth, wherever available. Wild greens from many plant families can be found, but the *mustard family* provides more tasty "relishes" than most.

TASTY MUSTARD GREENS

Latin Name	Common Name	Where and How Utilized
Barbarea vulgaris	Yellow rocket	Occasionally used as salad greens
Brassica campestris		California natives ate young leaves as greens
Brassica nigra	Black mustard	Luiseños of California ate whole plant
Bursa bursa-pastoris	Shepherd's purse	California tribes used seeds for pinole; whole plant as greens
Dentaria maxima	Big crinkleroot	Aromatic roots fermented then boiled with corn by Menominis
Lepidium sp.		In Louisiana, leaves were eaten as greens
Nasturtium officinale	Watercress	Iroquois ate plant raw with salt
Nasturtium palustre	Marshcress	Leaves eaten like watercress in Utah, Nevada, Alaska
Sophia halictorum		Pueblos cooked tender plants for food
Sophia incisa	Tansy mustard	Parched and ground seeds eaten by Indians of Montana and Oregon
Sophia pinnata		Several tribes prepared leaves by boiling or roasting between hot stones

TASTY MUSTARD GREENS (continued)

Latin Name	Common Name	Where and How Utilized
Stanleya species	Indian cabbage	Leaves boiled and eaten by many Western tribes
Thysanocarpus elegans	Lacepod	California tribes used seeds for pinole

These few examples by no means account for all edible flavorings, condiments, salads, and spices available in North America. Merely representative, these plants serve as reminders of nature's bountiful flavored gifts.

LIST OF REFERENCES

American Pharmaceutical Association. 1970. *National Formulary*, 13th ed. Mack Publishing.

Angier, B. 1966. Free for the eating. Harrisburg, Pa.: Stackpole Books.

Bailey, F. L. 1940. Navaho foods and cooking methods. *Am. Anthropologist, N.S. 42*.

Barnicot, N. A. 1969. Human nutrition: evolutionary perspectives. *In* The domestication of plants and animals. P. J. Ucko and G. Dimbleby (editors). Chicago: Aldine Publishing.

Barrett, S. A. 1952. Material aspects of Pomo culture. *Bull. Public Mus. Milwaukee.*

Bentley, R., and Trimen, H. 1880. Medicinal plants. (q.v.) London: J. & A. Churchill.

Beverly, R. 1947. The history and present state of Virginia. Ed. by L. B. Wright. Chapel Hill: Univ. of North Carolina Press.

Bodenheimer, F. S. 1951. Insects as human food. The Hague: Dr. W. Junk, Publishers.

Bourke, J. G. 1892. The medicine men of the Apache. *9th Ann. Rept. Bur. Am. Ethnol., 1887–88.* Washington, D.C.

Britton, N. L. and Brown, A. 1913. An illustrated flora of the northern United States, Canada and the British possessions. 3 vols. New York: Charles Scribner's Sons.

Brothwell, D., and Sandison, A. T. 1967. Diseases in antiquity. Springfield, Ill.: Charles C. Thomas, Publishers.

Burlage, H. M. 1968. Index of plants of Texas with reputed medicinal and poisonous properties. Austin, Tex.

Castaneda, C. 1968. The teachings of Don Juan. Berkeley: Univ. of California Press.

Castetter, E. F. 1935. Uncultivated native plants used as sources of food. *Univ. of N. Mex. Bull. 266,* [Biol. Ser., 4(1), *Ethnobiological Studies in the American Southwest,* no. 1].

Chestnut, V. K. 1902. Plants used by the Indians of Mendocino County, California. *Contrib. to the U.S. Nat. Herbarium,* 7(3). Washington, D.C.

Claus, E. P. 1961. Pharmacognosy. 4th ed. Philadephia: Lea & Febiger.

Coville, F. V. 1897. Notes on the plants used by the Klamath Indians of Oregon. *Contrib. to the U.S. Nat. Herbarium,* 5(2).

Cutting, W. C. 1969. Handbook of pharmacology. New York: Appleton-Century-Crofts.

De Laszlo, H. and Henshaw, P. 1954. Plant materials used by primitive peoples to affect fertility. *Science,* 119, (3097).

Densmore, F. 1928. Uses of plants by the Chippewa Indians. *44th Ann. Rept. Bur. Am. Ethnol., 1926–27.* Washington, D.C.

Driver, H. E. 1961. Indians of North America. Chicago: Univ. of Chicago Press.

Elmore, F. H. 1944. Ethnobotany of the Navajo. Univ. of N. Mex. Press.

Fernald, M. L. and Kinsey, A. C. 1943. Edible wild plants of eastern North America. Cornwall-on-Hudson, N.Y.: Idlewild Press.

Galinat, W. C. 1965. The evolution of corn and culture in North America. *Economic Botany,* 19.

Gathercoal, E. N. and Wirth, E. H., 1936. Pharmacognosy. Philadelphia: Lea & Febiger.

Gilmore, M. R. 1919. Uses of plants by Indians of the Missouri river region. *33d Ann. Rept. Bur. Am. Ethnol., 1911–12.* Washington, D.C.

Grimm, W. C. 1968. Recognizing flowering wild plants. Harrisburg, Pa.: Stackpole Books.

Grinnell, G. B. 1905. Some Cheyenne plant medicines. *Am. Anthropologist, N.S. 7(1).*

Harrington, H. D. 1967. Edible native plants of the Rocky Mountains. Univ. of N. Mex. Press.

Harris, B. C. 1968. Eat the weeds. Barre, Mass.: Barre Publishers.

Haskin, L. L. 1967. Wild flowers of the Pacific coast. Portland: Binfords & Mort.

Heizer, R. F. 1978. Man the hunter-gatherer: food availability vs. biological factors. *In* Progress in human nutrition, S. M. Margen and R. A. Ogar (editors). Westport, Conn.: AVI.

Henkel, A. 1904. Weeds used in medicine. *USDA, Farmer's Bull.* 188.

————. 1906. Wild medicinal plants of the U.S. *USDA, Bur. Pl. Ind. Bull.* 89.

————. 1907. American root drugs. *USDA, Bur. Pl. Ind. Bull.* 107.

————. 1909. American medicinal barks. *USDA, Bur. Pl. Ind. Bul.* 139.

————. 1911. American medicinal leaves & herbs. *USDA, Bur. Pl. Ind. Bull.* 219.

————. 1913. American medicinal flowers, fruits, and seeds. *USDA, Bur. Pl. Ind. Bull.* 26.

Hoffer, A. and Osmond, H. 1967. The hallucinogens. New York: Academic Press.

Johnston, A. 1970. Blackfoot Indian utilization of the flora of the northwestern Great Plains. *Economic Botany,* 24(3).

Josselyn, J. 1860. New England's rarities discovered. In *Arch. Amer., Trans. Coll. Am. Antiq. Soc.,* 4. Boston.

Krochmal, A. and LeQuesne, P. W. 1970. Pokeweed (*Phytolacca americana*): Possible source of a molluscicide. *USDA Forest Serv. Res. Paper NE-177.* NE Forest Exp. Sta., Upper Darby, Pa.

Lewis, M. and Clark, W. 1953. The journals of Lewis and Clark, Ed. by Bernard DeVoto (q.v.). Boston: Houghton Mifflin & Co.

Millspaugh, C. F. 1887. American medicinal plants, an illustrated and descriptive guide to the American plants used as homoeopathic remedies. 2 vols. New York: Boericke & Tafel.

Moodie, R. L. 1967. General considerations of the evidences of pathological conditions found among fossil animals. *In* Diseases in antiquity. D. Brothwell and A. T. Sandison (editors). Springfield, Ill.: Charles C. Thomas, Publishers.

Mooney, J. 1891. The sacred formulas of the Cherokees. *7th Ann. Rept. Bur. Am. Ethnol. 1885–86.* Washington, D.C.

Palmer, E. 1878. Plants used by the Indians of the United States. *American Naturalist 12.*

Parker, A. C. 1910. Iroquois uses of maize and other food plants. *N. Y. State Museum, Bull. 144.*

Platt, R. 1968. Discover American trees. New York: Dodd, Mead.

Quin, P. J. 1959. Food and feeding habits of the Pedi. Johannesburg: Witwatersand University.

Roys, R. L. 1931. The ethno-botany of the Maya. Pub. 2, *Dept. Mid. Am. Res.* New Orleans: Tulane Univ.

Safford, W. E. 1916. Narcotic plants and stimulants of the ancient Americans. *Ann. Rept. Bd. of Regents Smithsonian Inst.,* Washington, D.C.

Sandison, A. T., and C. Wells. 1967. Diseases of the reproductive system. *In* Diseases in antiquity. Springfield, Ill.: Charles C. Thomas, Publishers.

Schultes, R. E. 1939. The economic botany of the Kiowa Indians. Bot. Mus. of Harvard Univ., Cambridge, Mass.

————. 1960. Native narcotics of the New World. *3d Annual Visiting Lecture Series,* Univ. of Tex. Coll. of Pharm., Austin.

Smith, H. H. 1923. Ethnobotany of the Menomini Indians. *Bull. Public Mus. Milwaukee, 4(1).*

————. 1928. Ethnobotany of the Meskwaki Indians. *Bull. Public Mus. Milwaukee, 4(2).*

————. 1932. Ethnobotany of the Ojibwa Indians. *Bull. Public Mus. Milwaukee, 4(3).*

————. 1933. Ethnobotany of the Forest Potawatomi Indians. *Bull. Public Mus. Milwaukee, 4(3).*

Speck, F. G. 1941. A list of plant curatives obtained from the Houma Indians of Louisiana. *Primitive Man, 14(4).*

Speck, F. G., Hassrick, R. B., & Carpenter, E. S. 1942. Rappahannock herbals, folk-lore and science of cures. *Proc. Delaware Co. Inst. Sci. 10(1).*

Steedman, E. V. (ed.) (Based on field notes of J. A. Teit). 1930. The ethnobotany of the Thompson Indians of British Columbia. *45th Ann. Rept. Bur. Am. Ethnol., 1927–28.* Washington, D.C.

Stevenson, M. C. 1915. Ethnobotany of the Zuñi Indians. *30th Ann. Rept. Bur. Am. Ethnol., 1908–09.* Washington, D.C.

Stockert, J. W. 1967. Common wild flowers of the Grand Canyon. Salt Lake City, Utah: Wheel Wright Press.

Stone, E. 1962. Medicine among the American Indians. New York: Hafner.

Sturtevant, E. L. 1919. Notes on edible plants. Ed. by Hedrick, U. P. *N.Y. Dept. of Agric. Ann. Rep. 27.2(2).* Albany, N.Y.

Swanton, J. R. 1968. The Indian tribes of North America. *Bur. Am. Ethnol. Bull. 145.* Washington, D.C.

Taber, C. W. 1969. Taber's cyclopedic medical dictionary. 11th ed. Philadelphia: F. A. Davis.

Tantaquidgeon, G. 1928. Mohegan medical practices, weather-lore, and superstition. *43d Ann. Rept. Bur. Am. Ethnol., 1925–26.* Washington, D.C.

Turner, N. C. and Bell, M. 1971. The ethnobotany of the Coast Salish Indians of Vancouver Island. *Economic Botany, 25(1).*

Uphof, J. C. Th. 1959. Dictionary of economic plants. New York: Hafner.

1942. *United States Pharmacopoeia.* Mack Publishing.

Vogel, V. J. 1970. American Indian medicine. Norman: Univ. of Oklahoma Press.

Wheat, M. M. 1967. Survival arts of the primitive Paiutes. Reno: Univ. of Nevada Press.

Whitebread, C. 1925. The Indian medical exhibit of the division of medicine in the United States National Museum. *Proc. of the U.S. Nat. Mus.* vol. 67, art. 10. Washington, D.C.

Whiting, A. F. 1939. Ethnobotany of the Hopi. *Mus. of North Arizona, Bull. 15.* Flagstaff.

Wood, H. C. and Osol, A. 1943. The dispensatory of the United States of America, 23d ed. Philadephia: J. B. Lippincott Co.

Woodville, W. 1832. Medical botany. (q.v.) London: John Bohn.

Wyman, L. C. and Harris, S. K. 1941. Navajo Indian medical ethnobotany. *Univ. of N. Mex., Bull. 366.* Albuquerque.

Yanovsky, E. 1936. Food plants of the North American Indians. *USDA Misc. Publ. 237.* Washington, D.C.

Plant Index

English - Latin

Vetch, milk; ground plum (*Astragalus nitidus*), 109, 167, 168
Violet, dogtooth; glacier lily (*Erythronium grandiflora*), 185
Virginia anemone (*Anemone virginiana*), 27
Virginia snakeroot (*Aristolochia serpentaria*), 62, 128
Virgin's-bower, western; traveler's-joy (*Clematis ligusticifolia*), 62, 124

Wafer ash; three-leaved hop tree (*Ptelea trifoliata*), 121
Wahoo (*Euonymus atropurpureus*), 71
Wallflower, western (*Erysimum capitatum*), 124
Wapatoo; arrowhead (*Sagittaria latifolia*), 206
Water avens (*Geum rivale*), 125
Water chinquapin (*Nelumbo lutea*), 207
Water hemlock (*Cicuta maculata*), 42, 190
Water lily; pond lily (var. spp. of *Nuphar*), 206
Watermelon (*Citrullus vulgaris*), 205
Western clematis; western virgin's-bower (*Clematis ligusticifolia*), 62
Western hemlock (*Tsuga heterophylla*), 75, 195
Western ragweed (*Ambrosia psilostachya*), 58
Western virgin's-bower (*Clematis ligusticifolia*), 62, 124
Western wallflower (*Erysimum capitatum*), 124
Western wood lily (*Lilium philadelphicum*, var. *andinum*), 77
Wheat (*Triticum aestivum*), 183
White ash (*Fraxinus americana*), 111, 123, 128
White baneberry (*Actaea alba*), 8, 93
White beech (*Fagus grandifolia*), 63, 160
White cedar; arborvitae (*Thuja occidentalis*), 66, 90, 193
White clematis; western virgin's-bower (*Clematis ligusticifolia*), 62
White milkwort (*Polygala alba*), 55
White oak (*Quercus alba*), 16, 51, 72, 160–162
White pine (*Pinus strobus*), 39, 44, 129, 146, 197
White (silver) poplar (*Populus alba*), 60
White trillium (*Trillium grandiflorum*), 105
White willow (*Salix alba*), 61
Wild balsam; yerba santa (*Eriodictyon californicum*), 21, 97, 113
Wild bergamot (*Monarda fistulosa*), 29, 39, 124
Wild black cherry (*Prunus serotina*), 36, 50, 63, 121, 199
Wild black currant (*Ribes americanum*), 83, 200
Wild carrot (*Daucus carota*), 48, 90
Wild cherry (var. spp. of *Prunus*), 44

Wild columbine (*Aquilegia canadensis*), 19
Wild garlic (var. spp. of *Allium*), 76, 120, 185
Wild ginger (*Asarum canadense*), 42, 55, 71
Wild grape (*Vitis cordifolia*), 131
Wild indigo (*Baptisia tinctoria*), 16
Wild leek (var. spp. of *Allium*), 76, 185
Wild lettuce (*Lactuca canadensis*), 110, 123, 172
Wild mint (*Mentha canadensis*), 137
Wild oat (*Avena fatua*), 181
Wild onion (var. spp. of *Allium*), 76
Wild pansy (*Viola tricolor*), 27
Wild plum (*Prunus americana*), 96, 142
Wild rhubarb (*Rumex humenosepalus*), 39
Wild rice (*Zizania aquatica*), 182
Wild rose (var. spp. of *Rosa* and *Rosa speciosa*), 135, 200
Wild rye, beardless (*Elymus triticoides*), 183
Wild (American) senna (*Cassia marilandica*), 85, 108
Wild sunflower (var. spp. of *Helianthus*), 77
Willow (var. spp. of *Salix*), 47, 61
Willow, black (*Salix nigra*), 61
Willow, red (*Salix lucida*), 61
Willow, white (*Salix alba*), 61
Willow, western (*Salix lasiolepis*), 61, 124
Winter fat (*Eurotia lanata*), 64
Wintergreen (*Gaultheria procumbens* and *Moneses uniflora*), 38, 108
Witch hazel (*Hamamelis virginiana*), 73
Wood fern (*Dryopteris dilatata*), 64, 176
Wood lily, western (*Lilium philadelphicum andinum*), 77
Wooly groundsel (*Senecio longilobus*), 124
Wormseed (*Chenopodium ambrosioides*), 141
Wormwood (var. spp. of *Artemisia*), 30, 39
Wort, hairy umbrella (*Oxybaphus nyctagineus*), 32

Yampa (*Perideridia gairdneri*), 130, 191, 192
Yarrow (*Achillea millefolium*), 32, 55, 145
Yellow adder's-tongue (*Erythronium americanum*), 185
Yellow dock (*Rumex crispus*), 27
Yellow nut grass (*Cyperus esculentus*), 124
Yellow pond lily; eastern (*Nuphar advena*), 146, 207
Yellow pond lily; northwestern (*Nuphar polysepalum*), 206
Yellow root (*Zanthorhiza apiifolia*), 53, 96
Yellow-spined thistle (*Cirsium ochrocentrum*), 32
Yerba santa (*Eriodictyon californicum*), 21, 97, 113
Yucca (var. spp. of *Yucca*), 186
Yucca, datil; Spanish bayonet (*Yucca baccata*), 186, 208

Plant Index

Latin - English

General Index

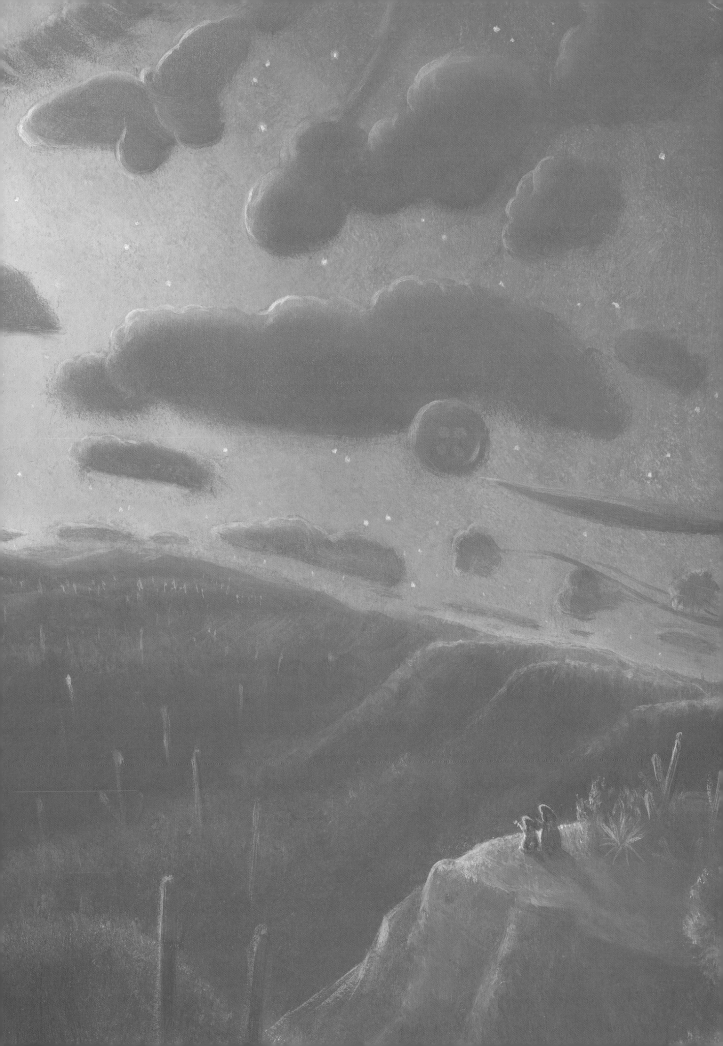

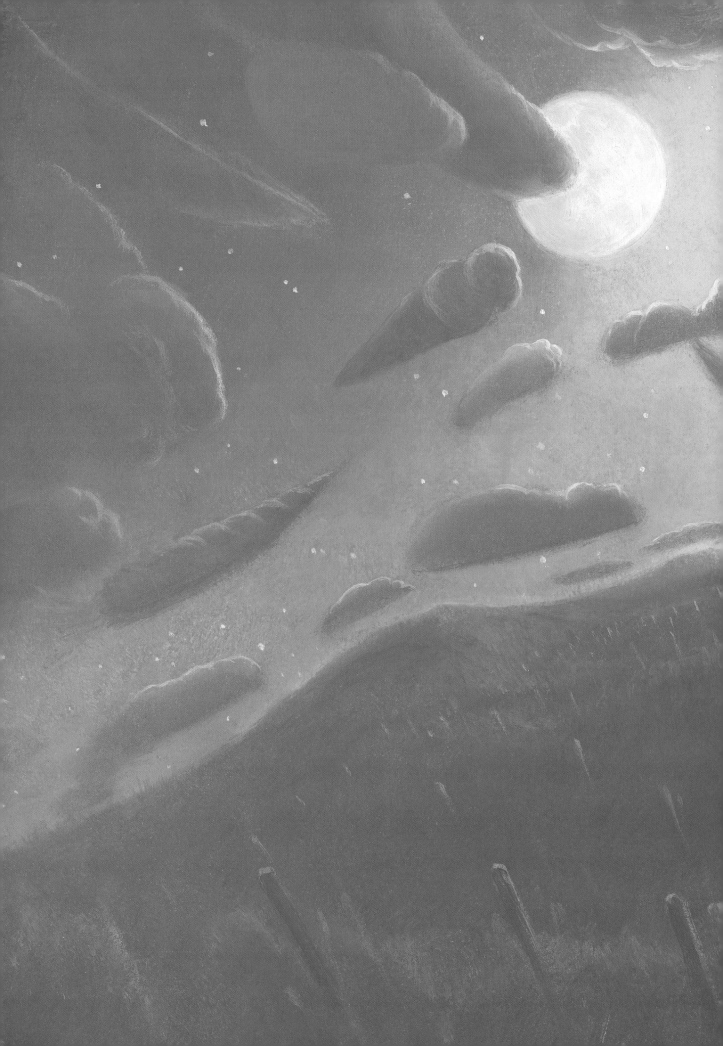

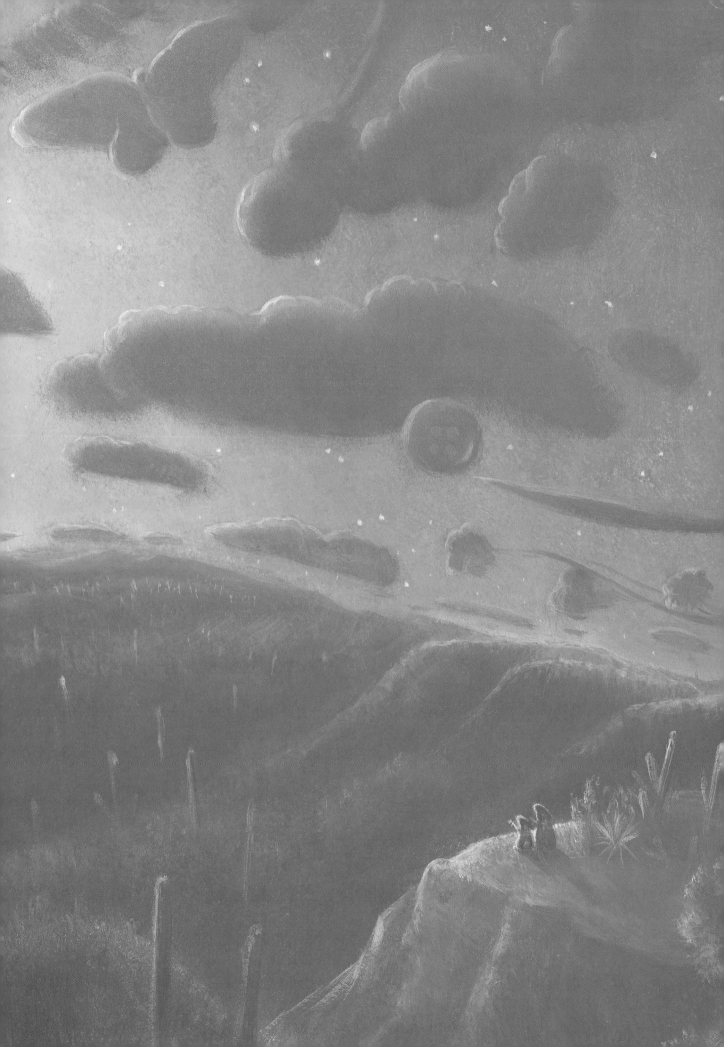

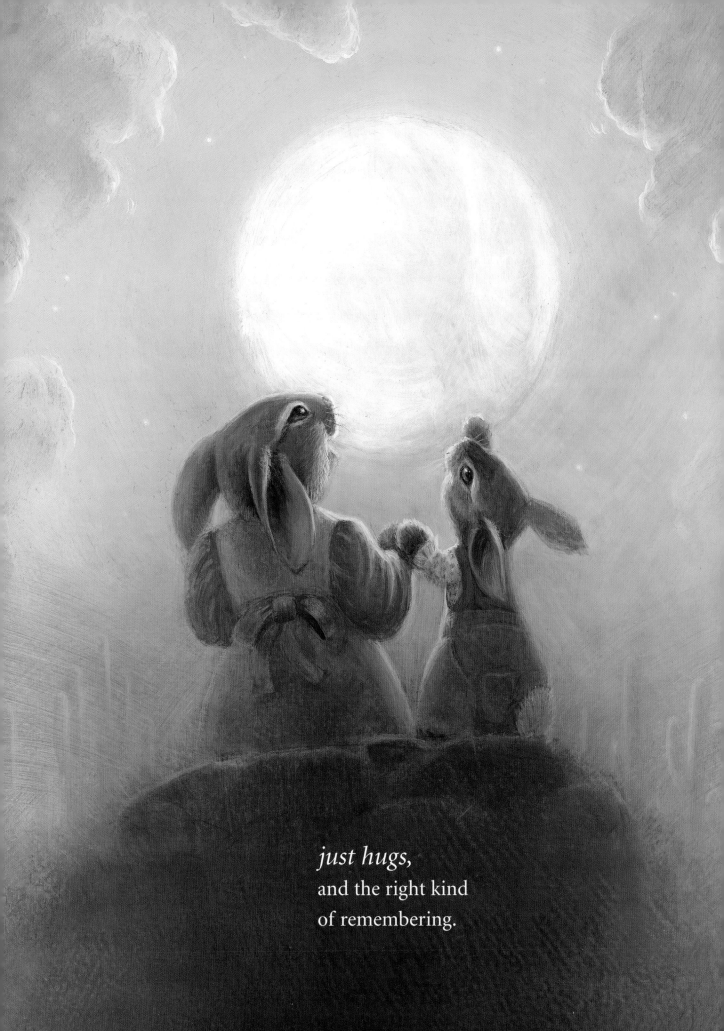

just hugs,
and the right kind
of remembering.

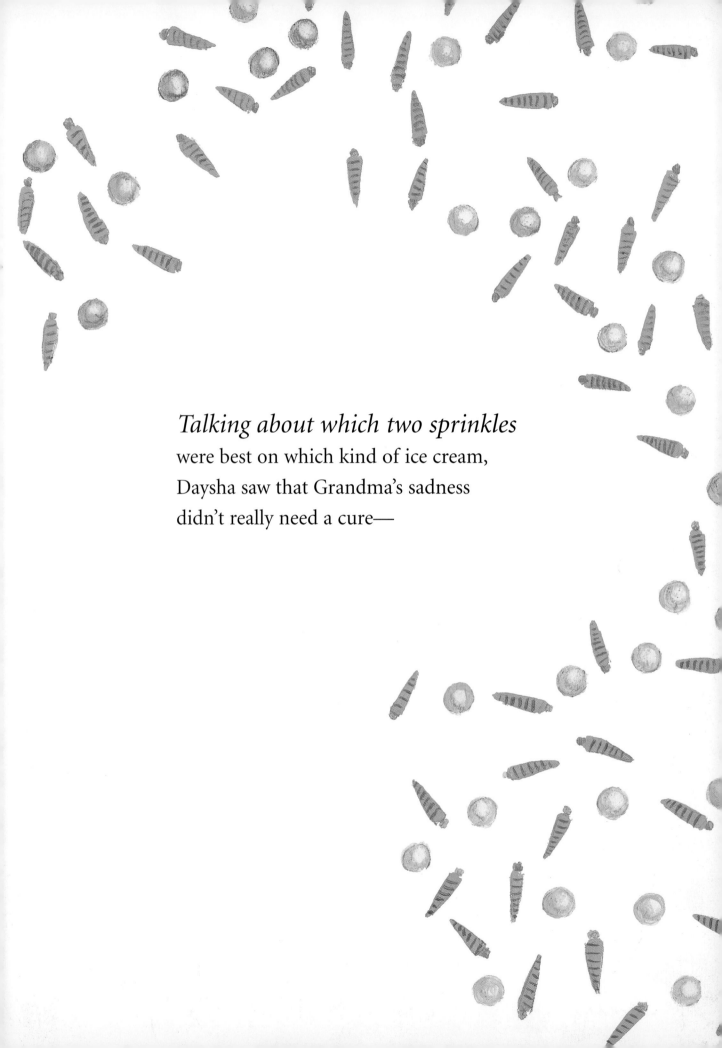

Talking about which two sprinkles
were best on which kind of ice cream,
Daysha saw that Grandma's sadness
didn't really need a cure—

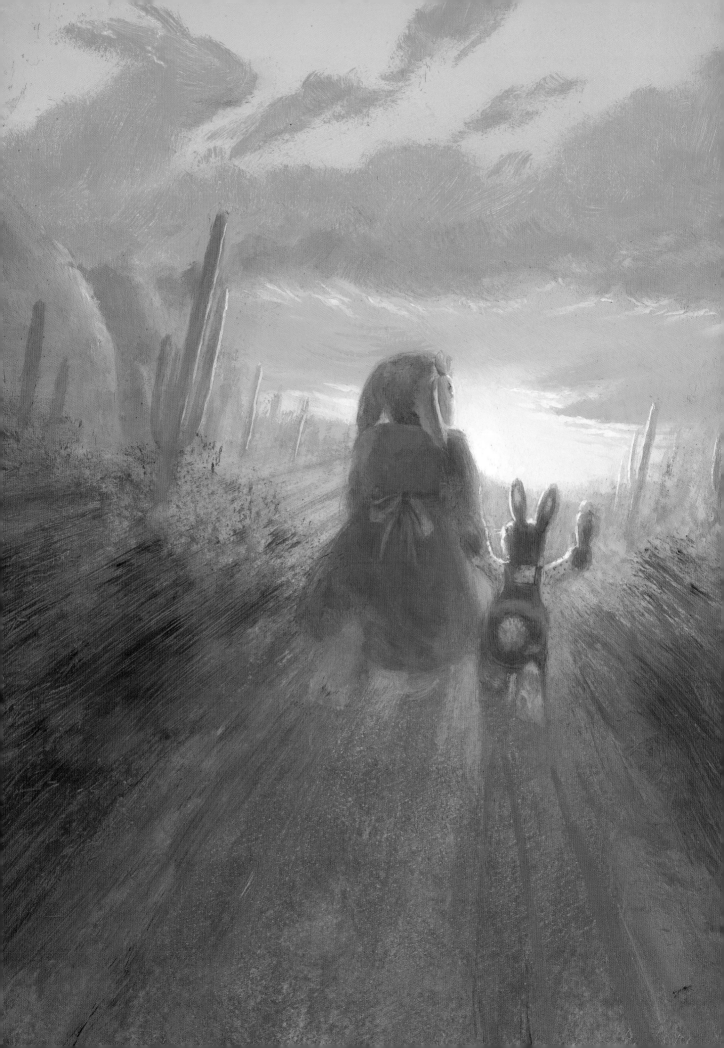

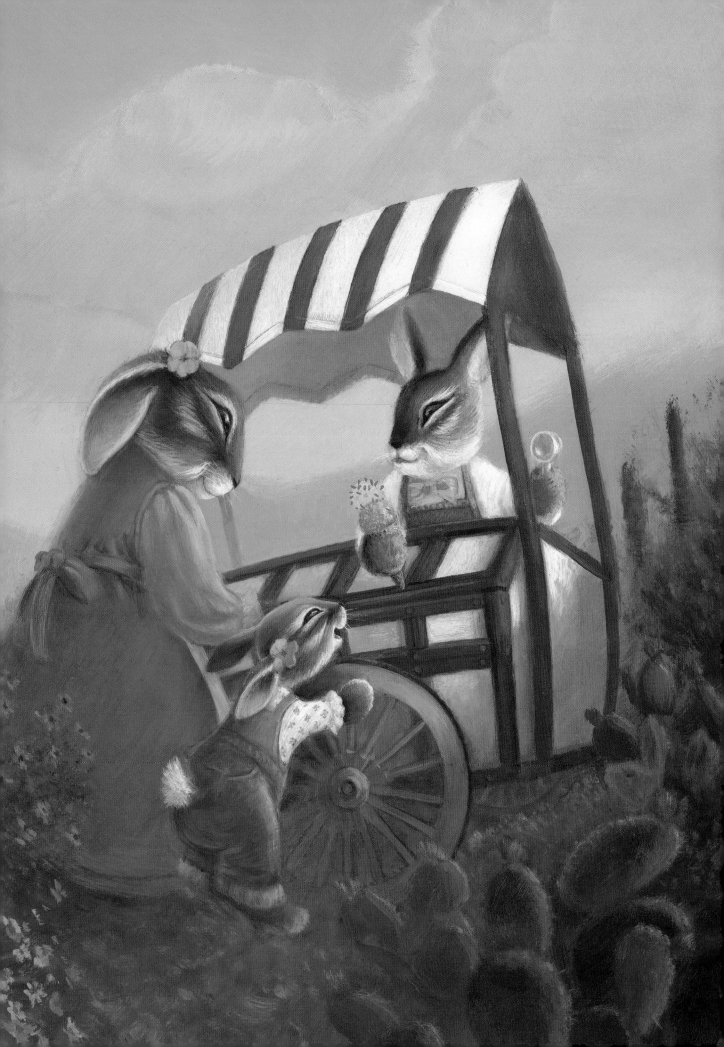